Also by Vicki Cobb

Chemically Active! Experiments You Can Do at Home
Fuzz Does It!
Gobs of Goo
How to Really *Fool Yourself*
Lots of Rot
Magic . . . Naturally! Science Experiments and Amusements
More Science Experiments You Can Eat
Science Experiments You Can Eat
The Secret Life of Hardware: A Science Experiment Book
The Secret Life of School Supplies
Supersuits

The Secret Life of Cosmetics

The Secret Life of
COSMETICS
A Science Experiment Book

Vicki Cobb
Illustrated by Theo Cobb

J.B. LIPPINCOTT   NEW YORK

The illustration which appears on page 99 is based on a photograph in the *Guinness Book of World Records* © 1984 by Guinness Superlatives Ltd., published by Sterling Publishing Co., Inc., New York, N.Y.

The Secret Life of Cosmetics
Text copyright © 1985 by Vicki Cobb
Illustrations copyright © 1985 by Theo Cobb
Printed in the U.S.A. All rights reserved.

Library of Congress Cataloging in Publication Data
Cobb, Vicki.
　The secret life of cosmetics.

　Summary: Briefly discusses the history of cosmetics and gives instructions for experiments which show how and why cosmetics such as shampoo, toothpaste, soap, and nail polish work.
　l. Cosmetics—Juvenile literature. [1. Cosmetics.
2. Experiments]　I. Cobb, Theo, ill.　II. Title.
TP983.C673　1985　　　668'.55　　　85-40097
ISBN 0-397-32121-X
ISBN 0-397-32122-8 (lib. bdg.)

4 5 6 7 8 9 10

For my niece, Amy Rachel Zabb

The author extends grateful appreciation:

To David Joshi, for his insights on soap and for review of the manuscript, and to Connie Meehan for providing historical information on soap and toothpaste, both of the Colgate-Palmolive Company.

To Harvey Koenig, for background on face creams, for determining the acid number for various waxes, and for reviewing the manuscript. To Paul D. Seplowitz, expert on fragrances, who also reviewed the manuscript. To Joseph T. Jakiela, for providing background on makeup and nail polish, and to Jane Cerri and Janice Corvino who put me in touch with the three scientists mentioned above, all of Chesebrough Pond's Inc. Research Laboratories.

To Dr. Mario L. Garcia, for reviewing the chapter on hair, and to Dr. John F. Corbett and Dr. Leszek J. Wolfram, all of Clairol, for information and insights into hair.

To Annette Green, of The Fragrance Foundation, for information on our sense of smell.

To Pamela Rosenfeld, my hairdresser, of L'Image, for supplying me with locks of hair, and to Philip Yablon, D.D.S., my dentist, for background on brushing teeth.

In spite of all the critical and professional assistance, the author accepts full responsibility for the accuracy of the contents of this book.

Contents

1. TALK ABOUT BEAUTY SECRETS . . . 3

2. SOAP AND TOOTHPASTE   7
    The Story of Soap   10
    Soap and Hard Water   12
    Soap vs. Detergent   14
    How Soap Works   16
    Acids, Bases and Soaps   18
    Deodorant Soaps   21
    Teeth and Beauty   24
    A Toothpaste Test   27

3. LOTIONS AND CREAMS   30
    A Barrier to Evaporation   32
    The Nature of Creams and Lotions   36
    Cold Cream   40
    Emulsion Stability Test   44

4. FRAGRANCES   46
    The Triangle Test   49
    A Perfume Story   52
    Extracting Essential Oils   55
    A Study of Perfume   62
    Perfume Staying Power   64

5. HAIR 66
   The Remarkable Hair 70
   Shampoo, Soap and Conditioners 73
   Curl 78
   Permanent Waves 80
   Bleaching Hair 81

6. MAKEUP 86
   Powder 89
   Powder "Wetting" Test 94
   Lipstick 96
   About Nails 98
   Nail Polish 100
   The Proof of the Pudding . . . 102

APPENDIX 105

INDEX 107

The Secret Life of Cosmetics

1. Talk About Beauty Secrets...

Walk down the cosmetic aisle in your local supermarket or pharmacy, and the message is loud and clear from all those hundreds of products on shelf after shelf. Television, magazines, and newspapers have been drumming it into our heads for years. "Buy me and have soft skin." "Buy me for brighter teeth and shinier hair." "Buy me and look beautiful." And guess what? People buy. Advertising definitely pays. But do cosmetics deliver the claims made by their ads? That's one question among many you'll be exploring in this book.

The word "cosmetics" comes from the Greek word *kosmetikos*, meaning "skilled in adorning and arranging," and has its roots in the word *kosmos*, meaning "order." (Yes, the word *cosmos*, referring to the order of the universe, is also from this Greek word.) But the term "cosmetics" has also been defined by law as "articles to be rubbed, poured, sprinkled, or sprayed on, introduced into, or otherwise applied to the human body or any part thereof for cleansing, beautifying, promoting attractiveness, or altering the appearance." Whatever it is that we expect from modern cosmetics, there are two things we can count on: the effects are temporary, and they have been carefully tested in laboratories for safety. Presumably, we are not at risk when we use them.

In the history of cosmetics, this was not always so. Cornstarch, once used as face powder, clogged the pores of the skin, causing unsightly blemishes that it then failed to conceal. Another popular face powder caused lead poisoning in the workers who produced it.

Cosmetics in earlier times were often used to disguise the effects of disease. Women once wore tiny beauty patches on their faces to cover the scars of smallpox. In the days of Queen Elizabeth I (sixteenth century) fashionable women wore "puffers," tiny wax balls they put on their gums in the back of their mouths, where they had lost teeth. The job of puffers was to puff out sunken cheeks caused by the loss of molars. Since they did not substitute for teeth, vanity undoubtedly prevented these ladies from dining in public. Until the last fifty years or so, when bathing became a part of daily hygiene, perfume was used to mask the smell of unclean bodies.

Today, many products are used purely for personal hygiene. Keeping clean is important for staying healthy, and healthiness is a standard that is now an important part of being attractive. When people think of cosmetics, they often think of makeup and

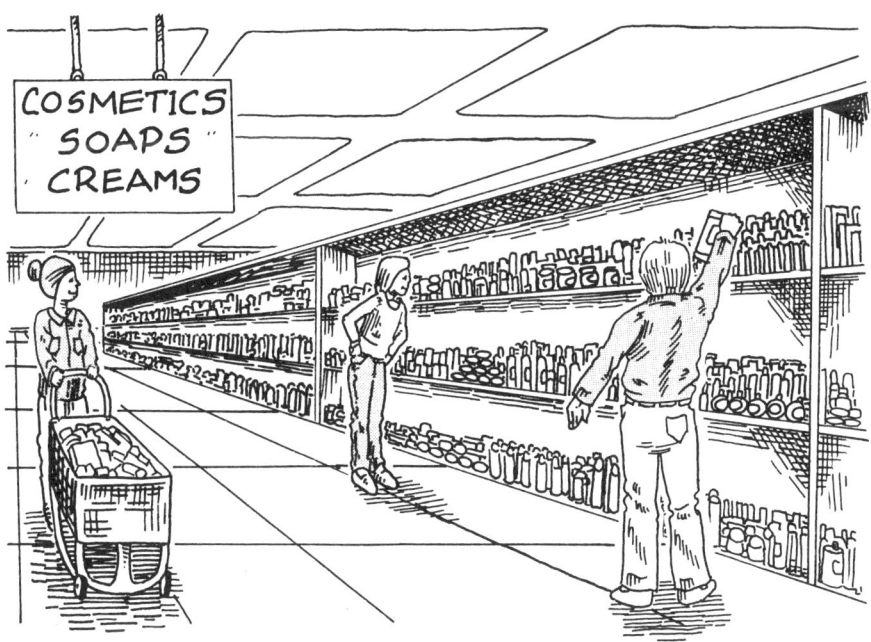

perfume. But the foundation of the modern cosmetics industry is made of unglamorous products for keeping you clean. Soap, toothpaste, and shampoo do an important job for your overall health and well-being.

If a healthy look is now part of what we think is beautiful, it wasn't always so. The notion of beauty has been quite changeable over the centuries. Women have been known to pluck out their eyebrows in one age only to darken them in another. At one time it was fashionable to be fat and pale, today thin and tan are in. But at all times there have been cosmetics. It has never been part of human nature to leave well enough alone. People love to fiddle with their appearance, and there's a booming industry to prove it.

There are many questions any reasonable consumer might ask

about cosmetics: If cosmetics do the job they claim to do, how do they do it? Is there a difference betwen very expensive cosmetics and lower priced products? What are the qualities to look for in a good face cream or nail polish? What is the science behind your skin, hair, and nails, and how do cosmetics affect them? I call the answers to these questions the "secret life of cosmetics." Cosmetics can be a fascinating subject for scientific research that you can do yourself. And if science is "not your thing," this book may surprise you. If you like to fool around in the kitchen, if you enjoy experimenting with cosmetics, or if you enjoy discovering new things about familiar products, get ready for an adventure.

Here's how to use this book. First, you can simply read it as you might read any book of nonfiction. I've included the principles behind each product and the part of the body it is used for without getting bogged down in details. Second, you can use this book as a how-to guide. I've included lots of procedures for testing products and recipes for making your own. I've done them all in my home laboratory and they work well enough to get you started. The funny thing is, doing something often gives you ideas for ways to do it better. So if you start wondering about ways to do something differently, go to it with my blessing! No book should ever be the final word for any creative experimenter from chemist to makeup artist. Trust your own hunches.

Cosmetics are partly dreams and wishes. But they are also real contributions to your health and well-being made by science. Discover their secret life.

2. Soap and Toothpaste

Good-looking skin is free of blemishes, pimples, sores, flakiness and wrinkles. It's something most people want, and they're willing to do some work to get it. No matter what else a person may put on his or her face in the hopes of producing clear skin, everyone knows that there's one basic rule to be followed before all others: namely, good-looking skin depends on cleanliness.

Our current devotion to being clean has only been in fashion for the last seventy-five years or so. Modern bathing became popular with the availability of modern plumbing. At one time, not so long ago, many people felt that the idea of a daily shower or bath was not only unhealthful but also immoral. They claimed that bathing was a sign of a declining civilization, and for proof all you had to do was look at the ancient Romans. After all, they were bathing regularly as their empire fell.

The Romans developed their idea of bathing more than 2000

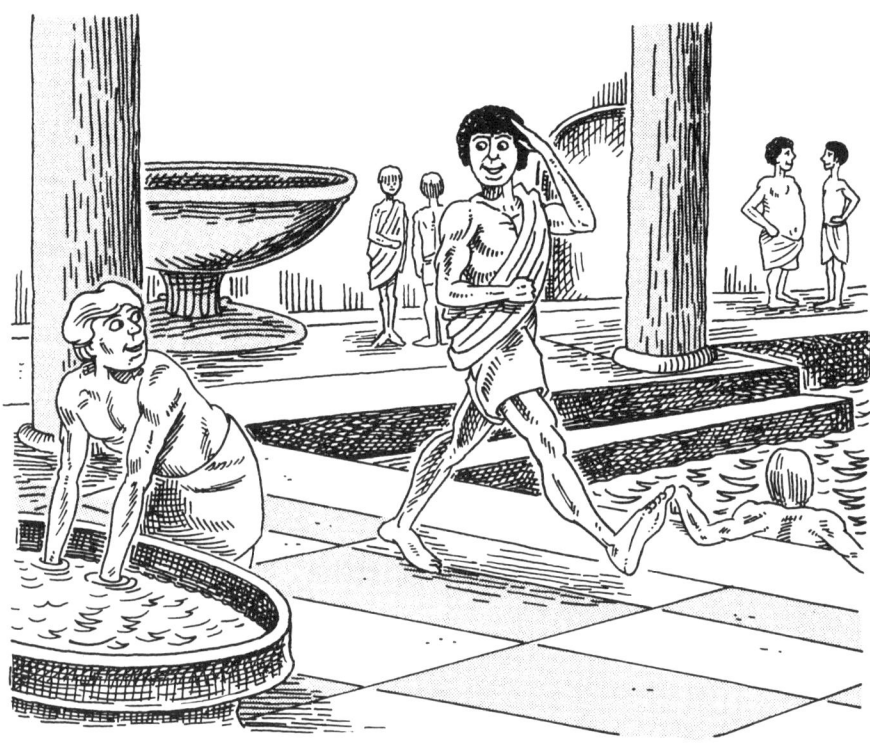

years ago from the ancient Greeks, who introduced public baths, and from ancient India, where steam rooms and the art of massage were invented. Bathing in Rome was not just to clean the skin. It was a way of life. Many Romans attended the public baths. A bell would ring about one o'clock in the afternoon, informing everyone that the water was hot. A customer would undress and get rubbed down with a mixture of oil and water. If he was really dirty, sand would be added to the oil. Then he would go to the hot room (like a sauna) to sweat out the dirt and socialize with others.

From there he went to the steam room, where his skin would be scraped with a special instrument to remove the oil, dirt and dead skin cells, and he was rinsed with hot water. Finally, he would take a swim in a large open-air pool. Afterwards, he might sit around in one of the meeting rooms of the bath, where he might hear a lecture or eat a meal. Baths in early Rome were for men only with special times for women. But during the decline of the Roman empire, the baths were open to both sexes. The Romans were so devoted to bathing that they built baths wherever they conquered territory. The Roman baths in Bath, England, are a popular tourist attraction.

After the Romans were defeated in war, bathing went out of style for quite a while. In fact, for some people any kind of washing at all was against their religion. One pilgrim boasted that she had not washed her face for eighteen years thus preserving the last water to have touched her face—that used for her baptism. Certain religious orders had a horror of water touching any part of the body but especially the feet.

Needless to say, a lifetime without bathing was usually very short. Death and disease were common in such unclean societies. But in spite of plagues and other mortal diseases, the connection between dirt and disease was slow in coming for the common people of Europe. Even among the wealthy, public bathing went through fashionable and unfashionable periods for hundreds of years. It wasn't until the middle of the eighteenth century, when churchman John Wesley pronounced that "cleanliness is next to Godliness," that personal hygiene started becoming a valued part of daily life. But until modern plumbing was made commonly available, bathing for most people was a Saturday night ritual at best.

The Story of Soap

One cosmetic item that most of us hardly ever think about, except when we run out of it, is soap. But when we go to buy it, do we ever have a choice! There's deodorant soap, soap that floats, soap that keeps moisture in the skin, soap for oily skin, soap for dry skin, pink soap, green soap, white soap and multicolored soap, some "soaps" that are not even soaps, soaps in all sizes and shapes, fancy and plain and, for the most part, extremely inexpensive. The choice can be confusing, except for one certainty: no matter what else a soap may promise, washing with soap makes us cleaner than washing without. *All* soaps give us that.

Soap, like bathing, also has a story. There are records from what is now the Middle East, telling us that people knew of soap as far back as 4,000 years ago. It wasn't the kind of stuff you're familiar with. It was an unpleasant mixture of oil cooked with ashes. But we can call it a soap, because mixed in with the grease and ashes was the chemical we know of as soap. This concoction was used more as a hair pomade than for cleaning anything.

Legend has it that the cleaning properties of this early crude soap were discovered in Rome, about 1000 B.C., when the melted fat from animals sacrificed in a fire for the gods ran down the sides of the altar and mixed with the ashes of the fire. Somehow this mess found its way to the banks of the Tiber River, where women were doing laundry by pounding the dirt out with rocks.

Lo and behold, they found that it was easier to get the dirt out with this stuff than without, and the first "miracle" cleaner was discovered. The place where all this happened was a hill named Sapo. So the great Roman historian, Pliny, gave this "barbarian confection" the same name as the hill. "Sapo" became our modern word "soap." The Romans used soap only to wash clothes; no soap was used in the Roman baths. Most likely because it was very unpleasant stuff that could severely damage the skin.

People knew how to make soap long before we understood its chemistry. Soap is made by cooking fats and oils with extremely poisonous and irritating substances such as lye, caustic soda or potash. In order to make sweet smelling, nonirritating soap, you must have exactly the right amount of one of these irritating chemicals for the particular kind of fat you use. Too much and the soap is grainy and strong, too little and the soap is greasy and doesn't clean or foam well. Early soapmaking became a business, with the best soap coming from the Castile section of Spain, where olives provided the oil for the soap. Castile soaps were used by the wealthy throughout Europe for hundreds of years.

In Colonial America, soapmaking was done at home. Lye was produced by mixing water and wood ashes in a bucket with small holes in the bottom and catching the drippings. Soapmaking usually accompanied the butchering of farm animals. Animal fat was melted and cooked together with the lye until the soap formed. It is a smelly and dangerous process (if not handled properly), which is why I don't include a soapmaking recipe in this book. The first American soap companies began appearing around the beginning of the nineteenth century. They took over this necessary and unpleasant task. It is no surprise that they were successful.

Soap and Hard Water

One way you know soap is working is from its lather. Soap bubbles form when soap molecules interact with water to form stretchable films that can hold air. But in some parts of the world, it's hard to make bubbles from local water. Such water is fittingly called "hard" water, and the hardness is due to minerals. Minerals interfere with the formation of soap films needed for suds. Water "softeners" get rid of these minerals. See for yourself the effect of hard water on soap in the following experiment.

Materials and Equipment
- epsom salts
- distilled water (optional if you live in an area where your tap water is soft. To find out, you can call your local department of public works.)
- measuring cup
- measuring spoons
- grater
- bar of soap (Make sure that the word "soap" is on the label.)
- waxed paper
- 2 large jars with lids

Procedure

Epsom salts are magnesium sulfate, one of the minerals that makes water hard. Put a tablespoon of epsom salts in one jar with a cup of distilled water at room temperature. Put the lid on and shake until completely dissolved. Put another cup of distilled water in the other jar.

Grate about two tablespoons of soap onto some waxed paper. Put ½ teaspoon of grated soap in each jar. Put the lids on and shake each jar twenty times.

Observations and Suggestions

In which jar do you get suds? Will additional shaking produce suds in hard water? Notice a white film forming on the top of the hard water. The minerals in the water react with soap to form this film. It's very different from the transparent soap-water film of a bubble. (Can you now explain the ring that forms around a bathtub?) Soap does not work well in hard water. So modern chemists developed a soaplike product that will. It's called detergent. More on the difference between soap and detergents later. Most detergents are used for dishwashing and laundry as well as body washing and shampooing.

Soap vs. Detergent

Do the following experiment to test different soaps and detergents.

Materials and Equipment
–epsom salts
–measuring spoons
–measuring cup
–small juice glasses
–grater
–waxed paper
–an assortment of soaps, including those listed as soap, as "bars" and as shampoos

Procedure

Dissolve one tablespoon epsom salts in two cups of water. Put five tablespoons of "hard water" in each of the glasses. Put ¼ teaspoon grated soap or liquid shampoo in each glass. Use a different glass for each sample. Cover the top of the glass with the palm of your hand and shake twenty times.

Observations and Suggestions

You should see a marked difference between the amount of foam produced by detergents and the amount produced by soaps. Detergents are usually not affected by the presence of minerals in hard water.

The amount of foam produced by a soap or detergent varies from product to product. If you would like to compare this aspect of soaps and detergents, follow the above procedure, only use distilled or soft tap water. It's important that you always use the same quantities of water and soap or detergent in every glass.

Another procedure for measuring the amount of foam produced

by different soaps was suggested by a chemist at a soap company. He said that foam would form on the surface of water if you dipped a bar of soap in the water twenty times. To make the test fairly accurate, there are several factors you will have to keep the same for all soaps. The factors you keep the same in an experiment are called the *controls*. You must use the same amount of water at the same temperature for each test. You must also have the same amount of surface area for each soap sample. Since the amount of water, the amount of soap, the number of times you dip the soap and the temperature of the water can all affect the amount of suds, you must control these factors. In an uncontrolled experiment you can't be sure that your results are due to differences in the soaps themselves.

How Soap Works

Your skin produces a certain amount of oil called *sebum*. Dirt on your skin gets trapped in this oil. Since water and oil don't mix, water alone will not remove the dirt. The water will roll off your skin, leaving the oil and dirt behind.

Enter soap, a substance that mixes with both water and oil. You can get the idea of how soap works by understanding the construction of a soap molecule.

Molecules, to jog your memory, are the smallest particle of a substance that has all the properties of that substance. Molecules are built of even smaller particles called atoms. There are ninety-two different kinds of atoms in nature, and each kind of atom comes from a substance known as an element. The main atoms in a soap molecule are carbon, hydrogen, oxygen and a metal, such as sodium or potassium. All soap molecules have a particular arrangement of these atoms.

One end of a soap molecule consists of a long chain of carbon and hydrogen atoms. During soapmaking, these long chains, called *fatty acids,* collect as fats, and oils are broken down. A fatty acid chain becomes one end of a soap molecule. This end is attracted to fatty and oily substances. It is the "water hating" end. The other end of the soap molecule has the metal atom. It is attracted to water and is the "water lover." When you wash, the water-hating end of the soap molecules stick into the oil. The water-loving end sticks into water. As the water moves around during the washing process, the soap molecules carry away the oil and the dirt that's in it.

Detergents work on the same principle as soaps, except that the fatty acid chain is replaced by another kind of hydrogen-carbon chain that generally will not react with minerals to form a film.

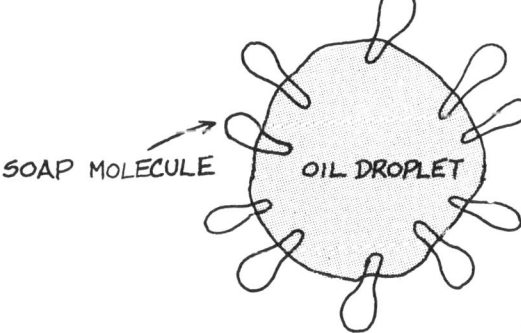

Acids, Bases and Soaps

Soapmaking is a chemical reaction. It involves bringing together two kinds of chemicals that form a new product (soap) when they meet. The two chemicals are an *acid* and a *base,* also called an *alkali.* Acids are typically sour tasting. Common acids around your house include vinegar (acetic acid) and lemon juice (citric acid). Most bases have a bitter taste and feel soapy. Household ammonia (ammonium hydroxide) is a good example. (DON'T, however, taste ammonia. It's poisonous.) Acids and bases can be weak or strong. Strong acids, like sulfuric acid or hydrochloric acid, are highly reactive and can be dangerous to handle. (Vinegar and lemon juice are weak acids.) The same can be said for bases. A strong base, such as lye (sodium hydroxide), can produce severe burns on human skin.

Since many acids and bases are poisonous and harmful to the skin, chemists don't taste or feel them to detect their presence. Instead they often use dyes, called *indicators,* which change color depending on whether they are in the presence of an acid or an alkali. One such indicator is litmus, which is pink in acid and blue in base. Another is *phenolphthalein* (fee-nol-tha-leen), which is colorless in acid and pink in base.

When an acid and base are brought together, they form a product called a *salt.* Interestingly, a chemical reaction between a strong acid, such as hydrochloric acid, and a strong base, such as sodium hydroxide, results in a product that is not only quite harmless, but essential to our health. That product is sodium chloride, or common table salt. A soap is a salt that forms from the reaction of a weak fatty acid with a strong alkali, such as lye.

When a strong acid and strong base react, their salt is neither like a base nor like an acid but is *neutral*. The same is true of a reaction between a weak acid and a weak base. But when a weak acid reacts with a strong base the salt that forms acts basic with an indicator. All true soaps are alkaline. Detergents may be alkaline, acidic or neutral.

Do the following experiment to test soaps and detergents to see if they are acidic or basic.

Materials and Equipment
–Ex-Lax tablet (your source of phenolphthalein)
–small square of waxed paper
–hammer
–rubbing alcohol
–heat-resistant custard cups (I have found that 4-ounce, heat-resistant custard cups are great substitutes for test tubes. I recommend their use in many experiments throughout this book.)
–measuring cup
–measuring spoons
–an assortment of soaps and detergents

Procedure
First, to prepare your indicator, you must dissolve the phenolphthalein out of the Ex-Lax tablet. Phenolphthalein does not dissolve well in water, but it does go into solution in alcohol. Wrap

your Ex-Lax tablet in waxed paper and smash it with a hammer. Put the powdered tablet in a custard cup and mix with two tablespoons of alcohol. Stir the mixture for a few minutes to dissolve the phenolphthalein.

Put ¼ cup of water in a clean custard cup with ⅛ teaspoon of phenolphthalein solution. Dip the end of the bar of soap repeatedly in the water. Count the number of dips you need to produce a deep pink color. Try this procedure on another brand of soap or "beauty bar." To test liquid soap or shampoo, mix about ¼ teaspoon of your sample in the test solution.

Observations and Suggestions

True soaps turn your indicator a deep pink. You will notice that some soaps turn your indicator deep pink with fewer dips than others. The number of dips depends on two things. First, stronger alkalis will produce a color change with fewer dips than weaker alkalis. Second, more soluble soaps will give a stronger reaction with the indicator than less soluble soaps. You will not be able to tell which of these two factors is producing your results in this experiment.

If you get no color change, you don't have a soap but a detergent. Detergents may be acidic or neutral and, as a result, phenolphthalein remains colorless.

Chemists and cosmeticians measure how acid or basic a solution is in a scale of numbers from 1 to 14 called pH. Neutral pH is the number 7. Acids have the numbers below 7 and alkalies have the numbers above 7. The pH of perspiration varies between 5.2 (fairly acidic) to 7.2 (slightly alkaline). The use of soap can change the pH of the skin. Since most of us don't react badly to soap, the change of pH on our skin is one we tolerate with no serious side effects.

Deodorant Soaps

The unpleasant smell of an unwashed body is due to the action of germs, or *bacteria,* growing on the skin. These bacteria use sweat and sebum as food. As they multiply, a characteristic odor clearly makes their presence known. A soap that is advertised as a deodorant soap should contain a substance that kills bacteria or retards bacterial growth. Do an experiment to find out if this is true.

Materials and Equipment
–one large baking potato, peeled and washed
–pot and cover
–4 custard cups
–Saran Wrap
–fork
–knife
–paper towels
–deodorant soap
–regular soap
–crayon

  Note: In any experiment where you cultivate bacteria, it is important that all of your equipment be as clean as possible. Clean, dry glassware that has been washed in a dishwasher is reasonably clean. Of course, if you want to be extremely sure that your equipment is sterile, boil everything in water, handle only the parts that will not be touched by your experimental materials, and avoid exposing your culture-growing material to the air as much as possible. If you follow these precautions, you can be reasonably certain that bacterial growth is the result of your experiment, not a contamination from unclean equipment.

Procedure

Prepare for this experiment by working up a sweat and not bathing for twenty-four hours. Put the peeled, washed, whole potato in a pot and cover with water. *Check with an adult before using the stove.* Put the pot on the stove and bring the water to a boil. Put the cover on the pot, leaving a crack so that steam can escape, and turn the heat low so that the boiling is moderate, not violent. Cook until tender, about twenty minutes. Test for doneness by inserting a fork in the potato. If it goes through easily, the potato is done. Turn off the heat and let the potato cool in the cooking water. This takes an hour or more.

When you are ready to do the experiment, slice the potato in crosswise slices about ½ inch thick. Put a slice, flat side up, in each of the four custard cups. Handle the slices as little as possible, and cover each custard cup with Saran Wrap. You don't want to expose the potato slices to the air. Mark the outside of the custard cups with the crayon as follows: control, water, soap, deodorant soap.

Dip one of the paper towels in warm water and squeeze it so

that there is still some water in the towel. Wipe one underarm once with the towel. Squeeze some of this water onto the potato slice marked "water." Immediately replace the Saran Wrap cover. Rub the same towel on ordinary soap, wipe the same underarm once and squeeze your sample onto the slice of potato marked "soap." Again, be sure to replace the cover as quickly as possible. Take the second paper towel and prepare it as you did the first. Rub it on deodorant soap, then pick up your bacteria sample by wiping the other underarm once. Squeeze the sample out on the potato slice marked "deodorant," and replace its cover. Put your experiment in a dark closet.

Observations and Suggestions

Inspect your experiment every morning and afternoon for the next few days. Bacteria colonies are tiny round circles that may be orange or shiny white. Molds are blue-green, white or black *fuzzy* spots. When I did this experiment there was an obvious difference in bacterial growth. The control, which had no underarm sample, remained free of bacterial growth for three days. The deodorant soap had a spread out orange growth but no small white colonies. The water and soap samples had many orange and white colonies. See if your results confirm mine.

It is clear from the results of this experiment that deodorant soaps do contain something that inhibits bacterial growth. The next question you might ask is: Does the soap kill bacteria on the body? Since most people wash soap off within a few seconds after putting it on their skin, the bacteria killing substance may also wash off and not be as effective as it should be. You could check this out by washing one underarm with deodorant soap and the other with regular soap. Then repeat the procedure, keeping the control and using plain water samples from each underarm. One would think that if the deodorant soap was effective, the underarm that had been washed with it would have fewer bacteria than the underarm washed with regular soap.

Teeth and Beauty

There is no question that your teeth have a strong influence on your appearance. A smile that shows straight, white teeth, with no spaces between them, is more dazzling than one of crowded, chipped and blackened teeth, to say the least. A good-looking smile depends, first of all, on keeping your own teeth, and that means keeping your mouth healthy, free of disease of both teeth and gums. Brushing regularly is crucial to maintaining good oral hygiene. (But it is no less important than maintaining one's general health and well-being. No amount of brushing will save your teeth if you suffer from a disease, such as scurvy, that loosens teeth and can cause you to lose them.)

Throughout history, the pattern of toothcare was similar to that of bathing. Some people did it, and others totally neglected their teeth, losing them young. The ancient Egyptians used false teeth and knew how to fill decayed teeth with gold and enamel. The ancient Romans cleaned their teeth but also used false teeth when their hygiene failed. But the champion "brushers" had to be the ancient Welsh, who kept their teeth clean and white by rubbing them often with a stick of green hazel covered with woolen cloth. They figured there must be some connection between certain foods and decay. So they did not drink acid beverages, such as wine, and avoided all hot food and drink.

There has been an almost endless list of *dentifrices,* substances used for cleaning the teeth. These included, at one time or another: ground chalk, ground charcoal, powdered pumice stone, soap, lemon juice, ashes, tobacco mixed with honey, a mixture of cinnamon and cream of tartar (ugh!), to name a few. During Elizabethan days (sixteenth century) a mixture called "Vaughan's Water" was a popular dentifrice. It was made by boiling vinegar, pine tar, spices including cinnamon, water and honey together, cooling the mixture and bottling it. It was more like a mouthwash than a toothpaste. Vaughan gave four rules for sparkling healthy teeth: Rinse your mouth after every meal (with his mouthwash, naturally), sleep with your mouth open, spit every morning and rub around your teeth and gums with a linen cloth "to get rid of the smell of meat and the yellowness of teeth." Toothbrushes were unknown, but toothpicks, often made of ivory or precious metals, were used regularly. If Queen Elizabeth I used Vaughan's rules for her own toothcare, it was not effective. Her teeth became yellow and irregular and in her last years were quite black.

In America, in 1877, William Colgate & Company, a soap company, helped usher in the age of modern toothpaste by manufacturing a dental cream. It was sold in a jar. In 1896, Colgate wanted to add a gimmick to their product as a way of making people sit up and take notice, so they put their dental cream in tubes made of tin. The instructions told customers to "press from the bottom," and a toothpaste "ribbon" would be squeezed out the other end directly onto the toothbrush. Toothpaste squeezed from a tube was a smash hit and was a major factor in encouraging at least some Americans to brush twice a day. But toothpaste for everyone didn't become a part of the American way of life until World War II. The armed services exposed the benefits of tooth care to millions of young men, who brought the habit home when the war ended. New types of toothpaste appeared on the market, many of them fads that came and went, such as toothpaste containing chlorophyll, toothpaste that was "ammoniated" and toothpaste that was "anti-enzyme." The only additive that has proven to make a major difference in tooth decay is fluoride. Somehow fluoride becomes a part of the tooth *enamel,* the tough outer coating of teeth, and makes teeth more resistant to decay.

Tooth decay is caused by bacteria that live off food trapped in the teeth. When you brush your teeth, you remove the food and some of the bacteria. Modern dentifrices contain a soft, abrasive substance that works like scouring powder, gently scraping the teeth without damaging the enamel, glycerine to give body to the mixture, a soap or detergent as a cleaning agent (obviously, one of the better tasting ones) and a refreshing flavoring.

A Toothpaste Test

Does brushing your teeth with toothpaste remove bacteria? Do the following experiment to find out.

Materials and Equipment
–one small baking potato, peeled and washed
–pot and cover
–3 custard cups
–Saran Wrap
–knife
–sterile cotton swabs
–toothpaste
–crayon or labels

Procedure
   This experiment is the same basic procedure as the last experiment on deodorant soap. But instead of seeing the differences

between the antibacterial action of soap, you will be seeing the effect of brushing your teeth on bacterial growth in your mouth.

Plan to do this setup just before going to bed, before brushing your teeth. Place a slice of cool boiled potato in each of the three custard cups. Cover with Saran Wrap to protect from contamination from the air. Wipe a dry cotton swab over one slice of potato. Re-cover the potato immediately with Saran Wrap. Label this "Control." Wipe the back teeth of one side of your mouth three times with a cotton swab. Wipe this swab twice over another potato slice. Label this slice "Before." Now brush your teeth thoroughly. Take the third cotton swab and wipe the back teeth of the other side of your mouth three times. Wipe this twice over the third potato slice and label it "After." Be sure to expose your potato slices to the air as little as possible. Put your covered custard cups in a dark closet. Check them every day for growth.

Observations and Suggestions

Did brushing make a difference? How sterile was the cotton swab? I found that my "Control" and my "After" looked pretty much the same. They were both covered with a light brown coating that may have been a reaction of the potato surface to the air. The part of the "Before" potato that had been smeared with the swab from my unbrushed teeth had a milky white patch. But the untouched area around it had the same brown coating. Bacterial growth had prevented the brown coating from forming in the center.

You can use this procedure to do any number of different experiments. When does your mouth have the greatest amount of bacteria, in the morning before brushing, during the day or in the evening? Do different brands of toothpaste have different effects on the bacteria in your mouth? Does mouthwash kill bacteria?

3. Lotions and Creams

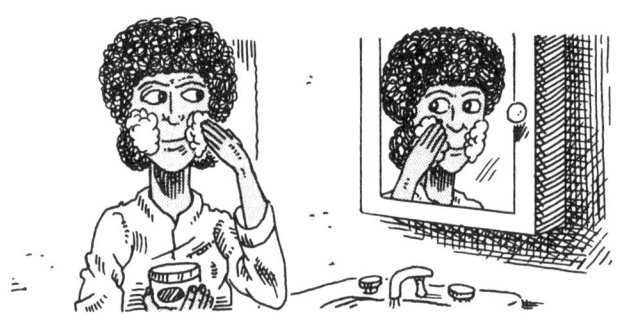

Your skin is a close-fitting, seamless bag covering the fat and muscle that overlie your skeleton and internal organs. It functions as a raincoat and as protection from harmful radiation from the sun. It keeps you warm and cools you off. You feel hot and cold, pressure and pain, hardness and softness, plus all kinds of more subtle sensations through your skin's sense of touch. Your skin prevents germs from getting into your body and it moves some body wastes out of your body. It is very much alive, constantly replacing itself as it is worn away or scraped off or cut open. In an average adult female, the skin takes up an area of just under two square yards, while the average man has a skin area of a little over two square yards. If you define an organ as a complex structure designed to perform specific jobs, then the skin is the largest organ in the body.

How the skin does all it does becomes more understandable

when you take a look at it at the microscopic level. Like every organ of the body, the skin is made up of smaller structures called *cells.* The cells of the surface and the area just beneath it are called the *epidermis.* The cells at the base of the epidermis are like small cubes. They are constantly growing and dividing. As they do this, older cells get pushed toward the surface. As these cells leave the area of growth, where they are nourished by the blood, they die and flatten out, forming the outside bricklike layer called the *stratum corneum.* The cells of the corneum are constantly being shed. But they are replaced just as fast as cells underneath move up, keeping the protection intact. The stratum corneum varies in thickness all over your body. Calluses on your feet are particularly thick stratum corneum. The stratum corneum on your eyelid, for example, is fairly thin. But, despite differences in thickness, the amazing thing about the epidermis is that it is really quite thin. The average thickness of both stratum corneum and the underlying living area is only $1/250$ of an inch.

Beneath the epidermis is a layer of varying thicknesses called the *dermis.* The dermis contains the base of the sweat glands and the sebaceous glands that make sebum. Both glands deliver their products to the skin surface: the sweat comes through openings called *pores,* the sebum through the opening around each hair. The dermis contains the blood vessels and nerves. The roots of all your hairs are in the dermis, along with the tiny muscle that attaches to each hair that gives you "goose bumps."

Most of the skin problems that are treated with cosmetics take place on the stratum corneum. Substances you apply that go beneath this surface and affect the generative layer, or dermis, are not cosmetics but drugs. Drugs must be proven safe and effective before the Food and Drug Administration (FDA) will give approval for sale. Cosmetics don't have to be registered with the FDA, but they do have to list their ingredients on the label. Some people have allergic reactions to some ingredients and the listing on the label can help them avoid products containing them. Drugs that are sold as cosmetics include antiperspirants, antidandruff shampoos, bleaching creams to lighten skin spots and sunburn protectors. Cosmetics such as skin creams and lotions are basically products for cells that are dead. Dead cells no longer receive nourishment from the body.

What can you do with dead cells to change their appearance? Get a piece of callous from the foot of one of your parents. (Cutting off a callous requires some skill, and if you've never done it, you can hurt yourself. Besides, older people have thicker calluses than younger ones.) Leave the piece of callous alone for a day. It will dry out and become quite stiff. Rub it with cream or lotion. You'll find that creams and lotions won't change its appearance very much after it has dried out. But you can see a dramatic change in the callus if you soak it in water. It becomes soft and easy to bend. So the most important concern of cosmetic creams and lotions is to keep as much water as possible in the stratum corneum.

A Barrier to Evaporation

One way creams and lotions keep the stratum corneum moist is by acting as a protective barrier. A film of cream prevents water in the skin from evaporating into the air. Much of the water in the skin is trapped in a protein called *collagen*. Collagen is one of the proteins that make up the connective tissue of the body, the material that literally holds all our tissues together. It is the single most common protein, making up almost 30% of all body protein.

Collagen molecules line up to form fibers that do not dissolve in water. Collagen fibers make up tendons and ligaments, as well as forming a network that holds skin cells in place. When collagen is heated, it breaks down and forms simpler proteins, *gelatin,* that do dissolve in hot water. When a gelatin solution cools, it forms a semisolid mass, or gel. The water in gelatin is trapped by a network of gelatin molecules in much the same way as water is trapped by collagen molecules. For this reason, gelatin can act as a "model skin" to test how well different creams and lotions act as a barrier to the evaporation of water. This is the goal of the next experiment.

Note: This experiment takes at least four days, if not longer. So it requires patience.

Materials and Equipment
–1 envelope of unflavored gelatin
–measuring cup and spoons
–boiling water
–aluminum foil or paper cupcake cups
–cookie sheet
–spoon
–an assortment of face creams and lotions
–Vaseline

–pencil and labels
–knife

Procedure

To prepare your moisture-losing "skin," put the powdered gelatin in the measuring cup and stir in two tablespoons cold water. Allow the gelatin to absorb the water. This takes a few minutes. *Check with an adult before using the stove.* Add enough boiling water to fill to the one cup mark and stir. The gelatin will fully dissolve in the hot water. Put one tablespoon of hot gelatin into each cupcake cup. You should have a cupcake cup for each sample of cream and lotion, one for Vaseline and one to be left alone. You are putting in enough gelatin to make a thin, even layer on the bottom of the cup about ¼ inch deep. Let it cool for a while.

Put the cups on the cookie sheet and place them in the refrigerator to set. It is important that your refrigerator shelf be level, or you won't get an even thickness in your gelatin.

When your gelatin skin is firm (after at least an hour and a half), you are ready to prepare your test. Smear ¼ teaspoon sample of each face cream or lotion on a gelatin surface. Use a different cup for each sample. Try and make as even a coating as possible. Label each cup to identify the sample. Leave one gelatin surface uncoated. This will be your control, as nothing prevents water from evaporating from the uncoated sample. Vaseline is the most protective material you can put on skin to retard moisture loss. So it becomes your "positive control." Put your samples back in the refrigerator. Let them dry for at least four days or until the gelatin in your control is a thin, flat sheet.

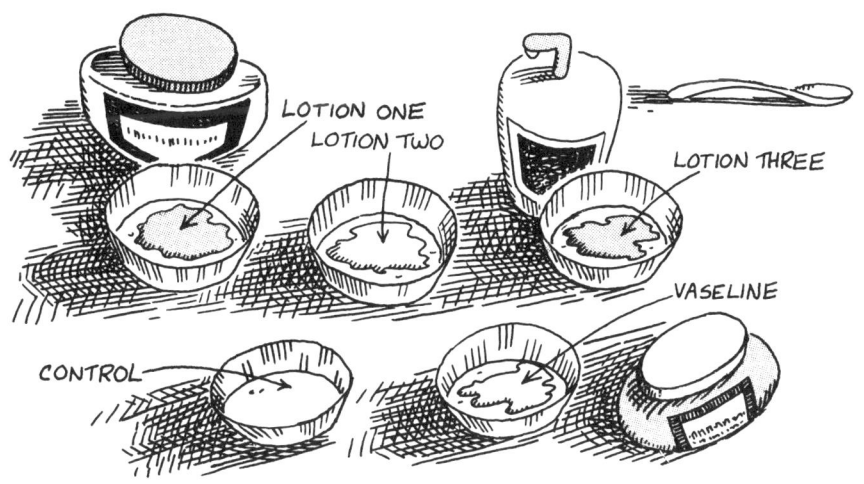

Observations and Suggestions

The thickness of the gelatin under each sample of cream tells you how effective it is in preventing water from evaporating. The gelatin that is unprotected will become a dry-feeling, thin, flat sheet. Remove each gelatin skin by slicing a strip through the center and peeling it from the cups. The thickness of the strip is a measure of how much water has evaporated. If you want to continue running the experiment, just put the cups back in the refrigerator. After a day or so, make another comparison by slicing off strips. Be sure to compare the thickness of the gelatin at the new cuts, not the old one that has been exposed to the air. Some of the creams will keep the gelatin moist and flexible. Vaseline is so effective as a barrier that it is often used to coat metal tools before they are to be stored for a long time to prevent moisture in the air from coming in contact with the metal.

Real skin is very complex. The gelatin film is a very simplified model of skin, doing only one thing that skin is capable of doing, namely holding water in a network of protein. Scientists often create such simple models in their laboratories before they test an effect against the much more complicated realities of nature.

The Nature of Creams and Lotions

Cosmetic creams and lotions are a particular kind of mixture known as an *emulsion*. Emulsions contain two parts, liquids that don't mix, such as water and oil. Many emulsions also contain a third substance that mixes with both, called an *emulsifier*. Everyone knows that any salad dressing containing oil and vinegar has to be shaken just before it is poured on a salad. Shaking mixes the ingredients for a very short time. As soon as you stop, the mixture separates into two layers with the oil on top. But if you add an emulsifier, which mixes with both oil and water, in the proper manner, water droplets can be spread evenly through the mixture so that they don't separate out. Mayonnaise is oil and vinegar salad dressing with egg as the emulsifier. Cosmetic creams typically contain water, oil, and soap or a similar chemical as the emulsifier. They also contain many waxy materials, which act as stiffeners or thickeners.

There are two types of emulsions. In one, oil droplets are suspended in water. This type is called an oil-in-water emulsion or O/W. The second type is the opposite: water droplets are suspended in oil, W/O for short. The feel of a cosmetic cream depends on which substance is doing the "enrobing" or surrounding the droplets. Oil-in-water creams are not greasy; they usually feel cool, and they "vanish" into the skin. Water-in-oil creams feel rich and somewhat oily. They sit on the skin and don't vanish.

You can easily tell if a lotion or cream is W/O or O/W. This and other properties of cosmetic creams are constantly being evaluated by cosmetic chemists. That's what this next experiment is about.

Materials and Equipment
–an assortment of lotions and creams including non-washable cold cream, moisturizers, hand and body lotion, suntan creams, lotions or oils, etc.
–a shiny metal spatula
–paper towels
–pencil and paper

Procedure
You are going to test various lotions and creams for different properties. So make up a data sheet as shown in the illustration on page 38.

To test to see if a cream or lotion is O/W or W/O, spread a small amount on a shiny spatula, add a few drops of water and try to smear the water into the cream. If the water mixes in easily, the emulsion is O/W. If the water beads up and doesn't mix in quickly, the emulsion is W/O. Another way to tell if an emulsion is W/O is to rub some on your skin. If it leaves an oily film that water forms beads on, it is a W/O emulsion.

Next test the "cut" or "peak" of a cream. Dip your finger in a cream and pull it out. Its there a long peak where you pull out your

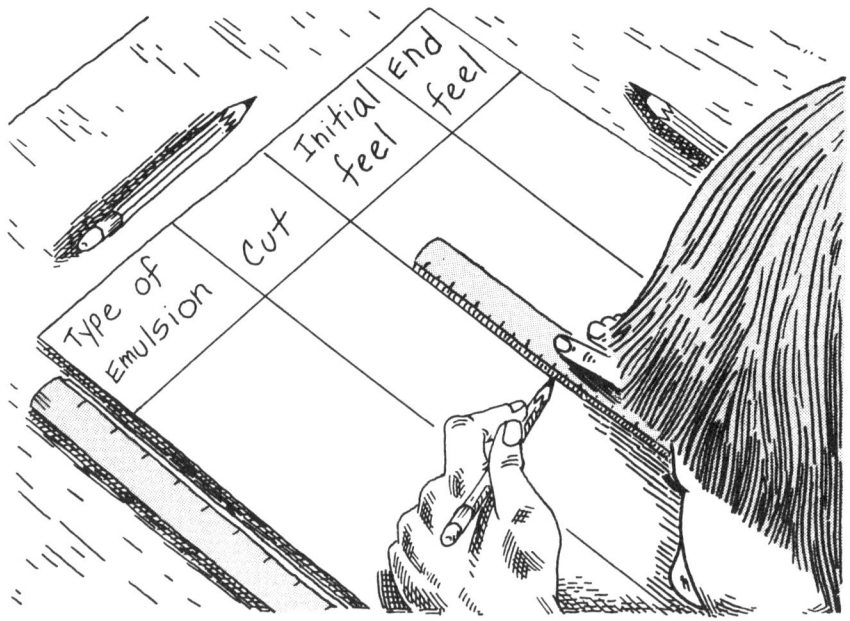

finger (or on your finger) or a short one? The peak is known as the "length of cut." You can measure it in millimeters if you wish. If the cut is too long or too short, it may indicate that the emulsion was not well formed.

Smear a patch of each cream on the back of your hand. Rub in well. As you test each sample, record your impressions of the initial feeling you get and the feeling after the "dry down" (when all the water in the cream has evaporated). Record your impressions on the data sheet. Here are some words to help you describe your experience: wet, greasy, tacky (sticky to the touch), talc-y (like powder), moist, silky, slippery. A word used to describe the cream that stays on the skin after the dry down is "cushion." Some creams disappear as if you never put them on. These have no cushion. Other creams are very noticeable for a long time after application. A cushion may have some "slip" to it or it may "drag." Both of these terms refer to the friction you feel when you massage a cream between your fingers. Slip feels easier to move, like an oil. Drag resists motion, and may feel sticky.

Observations and Suggestions

It should be very clear from this experiment that different creams and lotions have different properties depending on their jobs. A lotion that is to be spread all over the body usually feels more slippery than a cream that stays in a smaller area. A "vanishing" cream may have a tacky cushion. A cold cream feels greasy and leaves a greasy residue. You should be able to see a profile for each of the lotions and creams you tested.

When a cosmetic manufacturer develops a product, there is another kind of test that is as important as anything done in a laboratory. This is the "market test," with people who will buy the product. Cosmetic companies recruit people to try products and give them their opinions. No matter how well a particular cream does a job, it won't sell if people don't like the way it smells or the way it feels. Since a product test with people is likely to produce a number of different opinions, the results have to be interpreted, so that the manufacturer learns which qualities are likely to please the largest number of people. A special branch of mathematics, called *statistics,* is used for this purpose.

Since it is very expensive to get the opinions of thousands of people, between 300 and 500 people are questioned. This small number is a sample, representing the kinds of people the manufacturer thinks will buy the product. Such a market study will tell the manufacturer what percent of the people tested will like the product. Any test that has to be interpreted with statistics is less accurate than one based on direct measurement with instruments in the lab. But statistics are a useful tool when people's reactions to a product are an important consideration.

Cold Cream

Cold cream is a W/O emulsion that is stiffened with wax. Cold cream also contains borax, a compound that reacts with certain fatty acids in beeswax to produce a soap. This soap emulsifies the oil and water. Cold cream got its name because it feels cool when you spread it on your skin. This is because water in the cold cream is evaporating, and evaportation has a cooling effect. The cold creams you buy have many different ingredients. In the next experiment, you can learn how to make your own.

Materials and Equipment

Note: In this day and age it's hard to find pure ingredients, like beeswax. You need an ounce of white beeswax to make a cup of cold cream. I happened to get some at my local hardware store, where it is sold for waxing lines on sailboats. Some craft shops sell beeswax for candlemaking. An excellent source is a beeswax candle. Your best chance for finding one is a specialty store for candles, and you might also ask at some churches. I tried to make cold cream with wax products that are easily found in the hopes that they could be substituted for pure white beeswax. I tried a wax seal used by plumbers and a wax mixture sold in pharmacies for removing hair. Neither worked very well. Finally I discovered a reasonable substitute—bowstring wax for archery, found in sporting goods stores. Cold cream made with bowstring wax is not as creamy as the cold creams made with pure beeswax. But you can see the emulsion form, which is what this experiment is all about.

–a postage or kitchen scale (to weigh the wax)
–1 ounce white beeswax (or bowstring wax)
–borax (from the supermarket, detergent section)
–measuring spoons
–double boiler
–measuring cup
–spoon or whisk for stirring
–small jars for creams (use old cold cream jars or jars that contained marinated artichoke hearts)
–mineral oil (from the pharmacy or supermarket)
–boiling water
–paraffin wax (used for canning from supermarket or houseware store)

Procedure

Put one ounce of white beeswax and ½ cup of mineral oil in the top of a double boiler. *Check with an adult before using the stove.* Heat the beeswax and mineral oil over boiling water until the wax is completely melted.

Put ¼ teaspoon borax in a clean, dry measuring cup. Add boiling water to make ⅓ cup. Stir. The borax should dissolve quickly. Pour the hot borax solution slowly into the hot oil-wax mixture while stirring constantly. After all the borax solution has been added, remove the mixture from the hot water bath and continue stirring as it cools. When the mixture is warm to the touch, you may wish to add some perfume. A few drops can be stirred in. If you add perfume when the mixture is still hot, it will evaporate.

A smoother version of this type of cold cream contains paraffin wax. Put one ounce of beeswax, ½ ounce of paraffin wax, and ⅓ cup of mineral oil in the top of a double boiler. Heat over boiling water until all the waxes are melted. Put ¼ teaspoon borax and

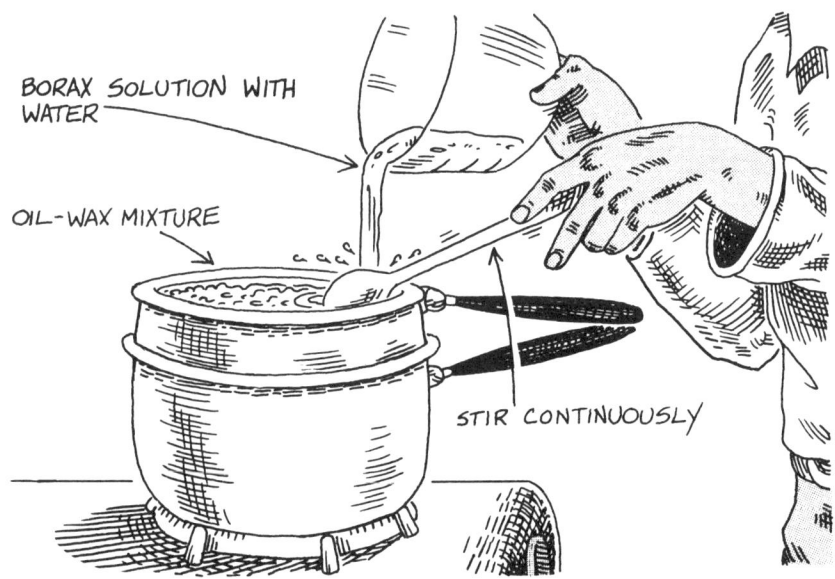

⅓ cup water in another small saucepan. Heat until all the borax is dissolved. Remove the borax solution from the heat. Pour the hot oil-wax mixture into the borax solution, stirring constantly. Continue stirring as it cools. Again, you can add perfume when it is still warm but before it is too thick. Pour into jars.

Use the following ingredients to make cold cream using bowstring wax:

- 1 ounce bowstring wax
- 6½ tablespoons mineral oil
- 3 tablespoons water
- ¼ teaspoon borax

Observations and Suggestions

The most striking thing about making cold cream is the appearance of white as the two clear substances meet and are mixed together. The whiteness is the emulsion forming as the borax reacts with a fatty acid in the beeswax to form a soap. Thousands of tiny droplets of water are spread in the wax-oil mixture and are held in place with the soap. Each droplet breaks up light, forming an opaque, white substance. An emulsion doesn't have to have a white look to it. If the droplets are small enough, as in certain hair creams, the emulsion remains clear. But when you make cold cream, the droplets are relatively large, and the mixture is snow white.

Test your homemade cold cream on the back of your hand. Test it against commercial products in the other procedures in this chapter.

Cold cream cleans the skin by loosening dirt and dead cells on the surface of the skin, which then can be wiped off. A thin layer of cream that is left behind makes the skin feel soft. Any oil that is used to soften the skin is called an *emollient*. Many skin creams and lotions are emollients as well as barriers.

Emulsion Stability Test

If the oil and water phases of an emulsion separate, a cream will obviously lose its appeal for a customer. It is very important that any cream or lotion sold commercially be very stable. The better known cosmetic manufacturers put their products through rigorous tests to make sure they can endure conditions of extreme temperatures. Creams and lotions can get stuck on trucks in freezing and in very hot weather. So they must be able to withstand cycles of freezing and high temperature without separating. Do your own test of quality control to see how well your creams and lotions hold up.

Materials and Equipment
–an assortment of lotions and creams including homemade products and off-brands (usually brand labels of the store selling the product)
–custard cups
–tablespoon
–crayon
–paper towels
–large skillet

Procedure

Put two tablespoons of each cream or lotion in a different custard cup. Label the cup with the crayon. Put the sample in the freezer. When frozen, remove the cups. Put hot water in the skillet and arrange the cups in the hot water bath. *Check with an adult before using the stove.* Heat gently until the creams are all completely melted. Repeat this cycle two or three times.

Observations and Suggestions

If an emulsion is going to separate, you'll see the oil sitting on top. The better known brands are all tested to withstand a cycle of three freezes and thaws. See how many cycles you need to make them come apart.

There are other emulsions that are not as stable as cosmetics. Try the freeze-thaw cycle on mayonnaise and on heavy cream. (Do not eat either food after doing the experiment.) How well does your homemade cold cream stand up to the test?

4. Fragrances

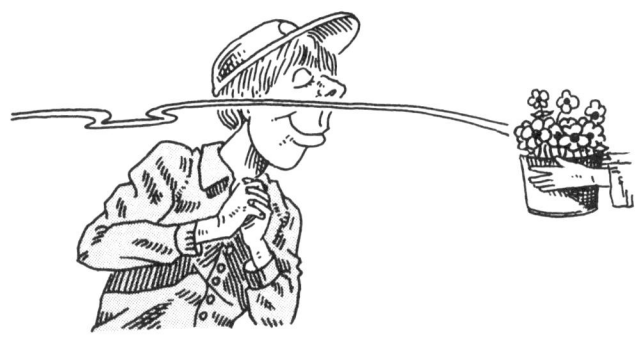

Smell was the first sense to develop in the animal kingdom. No surprise, if you stop to think about it. Animals that could detect food or danger some distance away had an advantage over those that couldn't. What simpler way than to detect molecules coming directly from the source? Smell is a chemical sense that detects molecules in air (or in water for water-dwelling animals). It helps an animal locate food or a mate and warns when poison or danger is present. For many of the simplest kinds of animals, such as flatworms, smell is the main sense for detecting things that the animal is not touching.

If animals can detect odors, it is only logical for living things to develop the ability to give off odors as signals. Skunks use a terrible odor as a weapon. Flowers give off pleasant fragrances to attract bees. The survival of many plant species depends on bees visiting the flowers. The payoff for the plant is that the bee spreads pollen, necessary for seed production. The payoff for the bee is nectar, a sweet liquid produced by flowers that bees collect and make into honey.

Smell, as a distance sense in human beings, has taken a back seat to sight, our dominant sense. But that doesn't mean that being able to smell isn't important. People who have lost their ability to smell find that eating is no longer enjoyable. Most of our sense of taste is due to our sense of smell. Have you noticed that food just doesn't taste the same when you have a cold? Smell enhances the quality of life. And it can warn us of danger, such as a gas leak.

In some ways, our sense of smell is quite sensitive. We can detect a skunk when there is one molecule of skunk odor in 60,000,000,000 molecules of air. Air and skunk odor move into the nostrils, passing under a patch of nerve cells in the back of each nasal cavity. Contact with one molecule of the potent skunk odor causes an *olfactory* nerve cell to respond. The olfactory nerve sends its message to the olfactory bulb, just on the other side of the bone that separates the nose from the brain. From the olfactory bulb, the message goes to the part of the brain cortex that determines emotions, creativity and memory. Here we decide that skunk odor is unpleasant. Scientists figure that forty olfactory nerves, of our ten to twenty million, have to fire for us to experience a smell. Since there are 250,000,000,000 skunk odor molecules in this breath, there's a good chance that forty will hit the mark. So, even when skunk odor is very diluted by air, there are still enough molecules around to make contact with our olfactory nerves, and give us a whiff. Dogs, however, are much better smellers than we are. They can smell skunk if there is one molecule in 20,000,000,000,000 molecules of air.

Our sense of smell is quick to tire. Lucky for us, especially when it comes to unpleasant odors. You notice a bad smell upon entering a room. After a few minutes, you no longer notice the smell. When you leave the room and then reenter it, you've given your olfactory nerves a chance to rest, and the smell is noticeable again.

When asked to describe different smells, most people are at a loss for words. There are no generally descriptive words for smell as there are for vision. You can find words to describe the appearance of a lemon to a blind person, but how would you describe its smell? All you need to mix any color in the rainbow are the three primary colors: red, blue and yellow. There are no primary smells. Nevertheless, most people learn to recognize about 2,000 different smells in a lifetime, even if they can't name them.

Scientists have attempted to sort different odors in various systems. For example, one such list says that the basic smells are flowery, fruity, spicy, resinous (like turpentine), burnt and nauseous (like rotten flesh). We have an excellent memory for smells. In fact, a smell can often jog your memory. The smell of homemade bread can cause a person to recall a pleasant scene involving homemade bread from his childhood. The perfume industry relies on pleasant smells to recall pleasant memories. There is, however, one thing all scents have in common: they are all *volatile*, that is, they all become gases upon leaving the surface of their source.

In this chapter you explore your own smelling ability, a way to make your own perfume and a test of perfumes around your house. Since this book is about cosmetics, we're interested in dealing with the nicest of smells.

The Triangle Test

Just as some people appear to be more naturally musical than others, some people are more talented smellers. They have the ability to detect the difference between two closely related smells and have a good memory for smell. Job applicants in the fragrance industry take a test to see how well they smell.

The test is called the "triangle test" because three sample odors are presented in each trial. Two of the three are the same. The object of the test is to name which two are alike. This is not a problem if the smells are as different as vanilla and coffee. But when they are closely related, differences in smelling ability can be measured.

The following experiment shows how the triangle test works. Discover your own ability and that of a friend.

Materials and Equipment
–coffee filter paper
–scissors
–sharp knife
–lemon
–lime
–spoon
–blindfold
–pencil
–a friend without a cold

Procedure
Cut the filter paper into strips about ¼ inch wide and three inches long. You need three strips for each test. With the knife, carefully cut off a piece of lemon peel and a piece of lime peel.

The next task is to transfer some of the oils in the peel of the lemon to the end of a strip of filter paper. The odor molecules are located in oil in the lemon skin. Place the peel, skin side down, on the end of a strip of filter paper. Press the peel over the strip with the back of the spoon. This squeezes out the lemon oil into the filter paper. Prepare another strip the same way with lime oil.

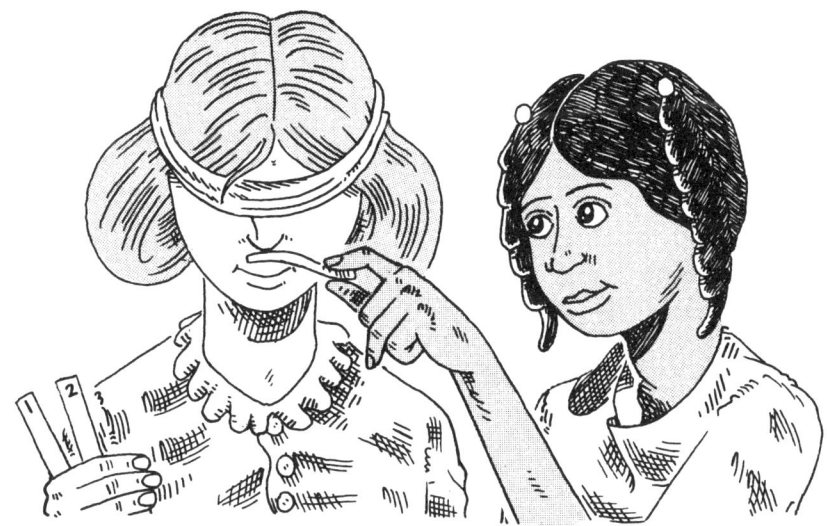

Make the third strip either lemon or lime. Number the other ends of the strips so that you remember which is which.

Blindfold your friend. Tell him or her that you are going to present three smells and to tell you which two are alike. Tell your friend the number, as you hold the oil scented end of a strip under his or her nose. One presentation of the three strips is a trial. You should do three trials for the test, alternating the order in which you present the strips. If your friend's sense of smell needs refreshing between sniffs, have him or her sniff a sleeve. Professionals take a whiff of their sleeves or of a tissue to clear their noses between the sniffs that depend on their judgement.

Observations and Suggestions

Did your friend have an easy time telling between lemon and lime? Try other closely related scents around your house. See if different brands of coffee have different smells. Try two perfumes. Test the difference between the cooking water of broccoli and cauliflower. Test the difference between apricots and nectarines, between almond extract and cherry extract. Try different perfumes, lotions and face creams. Do the triangle test on members of your family. Whose sense of smell is sharper—men's or women's? Science has suggested that women are better smellers. Do your results confirm this?

A Perfume Story

People first began to purposefully change the smell around them when they burned pine resin and fragrant woods, like sandalwood, as incense during religious ceremonies thousands of years ago. Fragrant smoke was thought of as a way to please the gods. Incense was burned in sickrooms to mask the smells of illness and drive away the evil spirits. So, it's no surprise that the word "perfume" means "through smoke."

The ancient Egyptians probably were the first people to apply fragrant mixtures to the skin. Some Egyptian may have thrown some flowers into the oil used at the baths and discovered how much more pleasing it was when the oil smelled like roses. The first modern perfume, a fragrant oil dissolved in alcohol, was created for Queen Elizabeth of Hungary in the fourteenth century. Such a mixture was only for the aristocrats. But that didn't mean ordinary folk weren't interested in sweet smells. During the Middle Ages and the Renaissance, sweet smells had an extremely important job to do—masking foul and unpleasant odors. People wore scented balls of wax, called "pomanders," on strings around their necks to mask the smell of unwashed bodies, as well as to ward off infection. They carried scented handkerchiefs that could be quickly brought to the nose in case they passed an open sewer. The practice of covering a casket with flowers at funerals helped mask the smell of a rotting corpse. Scent bags of lavender and iris root were sewn into clothing for freshness before the age of dry cleaning. Needless to say, the world did not smell like a rose.

Today it seems as if almost everything we buy, from paint to detergent to cleaning solution to inks, smells good. That's because smell has proven to be an important factor in the marketplace.

Given a choice between a foam rubber pillow that smells like foam rubber and one that smells like lemons, the consumer may go for the lemon pillow and may not even consciously know why. As a result, the fragrance industry makes an important contribution to many other manufacturers, as well as to cosmetics.

But the best smells of all come from the fine perfume manufacturers. The more expensive perfumes are a blend of between 200 and 500 different ingredients, some of them only traces. The person who creates a great perfume is not only a talented smeller but also a well-educated one, trained to tell the differences between hundreds of fragrances and fragrance blends. This high-paying and important job is held by someone called the "nose." Legendary noses have been known to not only tell the difference between different rose oils, but where the roses came from, when they were grown, and where the oils were processed.

I hold the deepest respect for a nose. Let me tell you why. Once I belonged to an organization that wanted to sell something at our convention. We had heard that the recipe for "Edelweiss" perfume in a book called *Henley's Formulas* was none other than the recipe for "Joy" perfume, once advertised as "the most expensive perfume in the world." So, we bought the ingredients at a specialty shop that carried fragrances and flavorings and proceeded to adapt the recipe and make our own version of Joy to sell at the convention. We made it in my kitchen, called it "Pure Joy," and put it in ¼ ounce bottles that were shaped just like the bottles Joy came in. "Pure Joy" sold for about three dollars a bottle, considerably less than the more than sixty dollars charged for the same amount of Joy.

Did our perfume smell like the real thing? Not really. When we were mixing the perfume we had a sample of Joy that we used as a standard. We all took turns sniffing Joy, trying to compare it to our mixture. We sniffed all the different ingredients to decide what to add more of and wound up thoroughly confused. After a while, everything smelled the same. I have no doubt that a professional nose would have laughed at our efforts and wondered how we could dare to think that a bunch of amateurs could even begin to create a fragrance that rivaled one of the best in the world. Nevertheless, we quickly sold out of the few hundred bottles we made, the newspapers wrote up our story and we never got a single complaint from any one of our customers.

For fun, in case you ever get the chance to try making "Pure Joy," I include the recipe for Edelweiss in the Appendix at the back of the book.

Extracting Essential Oils

If you rub yourself with rose petals, will you smell like a rose? The answer is not very strongly and not for very long. Hardly worth destroying a beautiful blossom, if you've got one. Besides, roses are not always available. We need perfume to smell like a rose or any other flower, spice or herb on a daily basis. Clearly, the problem is to get the fragrance-causing chemicals out of the source.

The molecules that make up most fragrances are not simple, like molecules of water and salt. They contain various arrangements of carbon atoms, along with hydrogen and oxygen. Other elements may also be involved. The chemistry of odors still is not completely understood. One modern theory of smell states that it is the shape of a molecule that determines its smell.

Not all fragrant compounds are natural. Chemists have synthesized some of the common fragrances in laboratories. But whether they are man-made or natural, most fragrant compounds do not dissolve well in water. They do, however, dissolve in fat. So fat is a key to extracting the essence of an aroma known as an "essential oil." Once an essential oil is in the fat, it can be extracted by dissolving it in alcohol.

There are several ways to extract essential oils from flowers and herbs. A cold method, called "enfleurage," involves sandwiching flower petals between sheets of glass smeared with lard. The glass sheets are piled on top of each other; thus the weight also helps press out the oils. This method has been used chiefly for roses. The essential oil, or *attar*, seeps from the petals into the fat. Enfleurage is a slow process. Every day for several weeks, the old petals have to be removed and replaced with fresh petals. The flowers must be extremely fresh, as cut roses quickly lose their ability to produce fragrance. The attar produced this way is of the highest quality. It is also extremely expensive. In fact, enfleurage is rarely used anymore. Scientists have devised other ways to get better yields from the petals and have learned ways to handle petals more gently so that the flower odors remain true.

The next experiment is a hot method for extracting essential oils. Heat makes essential oils dissolve into the fat more quickly, but it also causes some of the essential oils to evaporate into the air. This procedure is fairly ambitious. *You will need an adult with you to do the distillation.* You have to make a piece of apparatus. But once you've learned how, this procedure lends itself to many experiments.

Materials and Equipment
- 2½ feet of ³⁄₁₆ inch copper tubing (from a good hardware store or plumbing supply store)
- a large mayonnaise jar with lid
- a large nail
- hammer
- broomstick
- plastic clay
- heavy saucepan large enough for the jar to fit into
- lard
- ethyl alcohol (Vodka is the best source. Make sure you have your parents' permission to use it. Don't use rubbing alcohol. It has too strong a smell.)
- two lemons
- fine grater
- waxed paper
- potholder
- measuring spoons
- small glass

Procedure

The first thing you must do is prepare your apparatus. You will be separating the alcohol and the essential oils from the lard by *distillation*. Alcohol boils at a lower temperature than fat. When boiling, it leaves the mixture as a gas. When you distill something

58 / The Secret Life of Cosmetics

you trap the gas and cool it back into a liquid. The piece of apparatus that cools the gas is called a *condenser*. Your condenser will be made of the copper tubing.

The copper tubing has to be bent into the shape shown in the picture. You can get a nice spiral by wrapping the tubing around a broomstick. Get an adult to help you if you aren't strong enough. Start wrapping the tubing around the broomstick about two inches from one end, make five turns and bend the remaining length of about eight inches as shown.

Make a hole with the hammer and nail in the center of the lid of the jar. The hole should be just large enough so that the copper tubing fits in snugly.

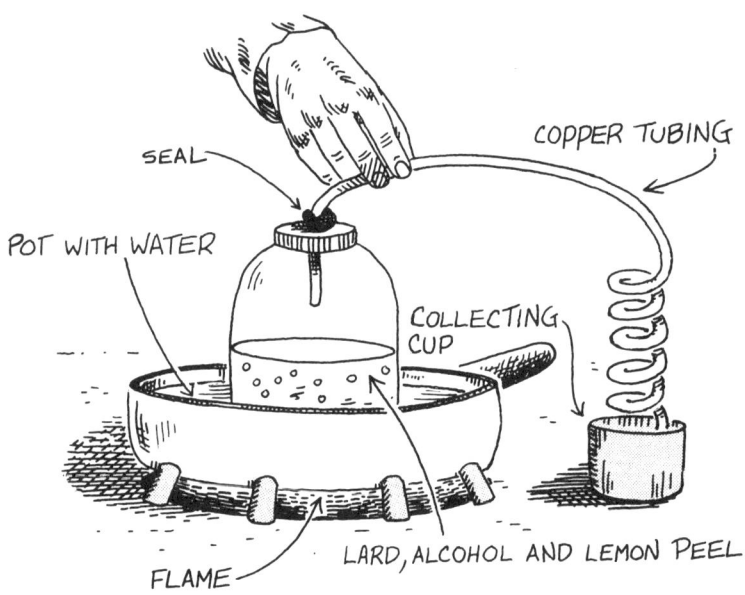

Set up your distilling apparatus and make sure that it's stable. This may take some improvising. The jar is going to be in the pan on the stove. The long end of the condenser is inserted in the hole in the jar cover. A small glass is placed under the other end near the coil. The biggest danger is that your apparatus will fall apart when you are heating it. So make sure that the setup is stable and won't fall over. The jar will be in boiling water and the movement of the water may move it slightly. *When you actually begin distilling, have an adult present to make sure that the condenser won't move the glass so much that it falls.*

Now prepare your raw material, lemon peel. When you want to extract the essential oils from a solid source, such as wood or seeds, they should be as finely divided as possible. Grated lemon peel has much more surface area for releasing the oils than lemon peel strips. So grate the peels off both lemons onto some waxed paper.

Check with an adult before you use the stove. Put ¼ pound of lard into the jar. Set the jar in the pan and add water. Over a low flame, heat the water bath until all the lard is melted. Add the grated lemon peel to the lard. Cover the hole in the lid of the jar with some plastic clay. Using a potholder, remove the jar from the water bath and screw on the lid. Again using the potholder, swirl the jar for a few minutes to thoroughly mix the lemon peel and the lard. Set the jar back in the water bath. Bring the water to a boil and immediately turn off the heat. Let the mixture sit in the hot water for an hour.

By now, much of the lemon oil is dissolved in the lard. Next you add alcohol. The lemon oil in fat will now dissolve into the alcohol. Make sure the alcohol is room temperature. Put two tablespoons of alcohol into the jar. Cover and shake for five minutes.

Remove the clay stopper in the lid. Set up your distillation apparatus, and make sure it is stable. Make sure that the water in the pan is at least one inch deep around the sides of the jar. *Have an adult with you before you begin distilling.* Turn on the heat. Keep an eye on your setup so that there are no accidents and so that the water does not boil off. Be careful not to touch the copper tubing, as it may be hot. When the water level gets low, add more. It will take about fifteen or twenty minutes for drops of lemon scent to come out the coiled end of your condenser into the glass. You should be able to recover at least half an ounce of lemon scent. Keep your perfume in a tightly stoppered bottle.

Observations and Suggestions

Can you smell the lemon in your perfume? Put some on your skin and let the alcohol dry. The lemon scent should remain behind.

Here's how the condenser works. The essential oils and alcohol become a gas leaving the liquid surface. Gas molecules travel into the copper tubing. Since copper is a metal, it is a good conductor of heat. The copper removes heat from the gas inside the tube and conducts the heat into the air. The tube is long enough to cool the gas until it condenses into a liquid. The shape of the condenser makes it more compact and allows gravity to move the drops of liquid into the glass.

This setup can be used to extract the essential oils from all kinds of sources, including flowers. The rule is that ¼ pound of lard will absorb the oil from ¾ pound of flowers. Since you cannot put all the flowers in at once, you will have to extract the essential oils in stages. Fill the jar over the melted lard with flowers that have been freshly picked and have no stems. Shake well to coat the petals with melted fat. Let stand for an hour. Strain the fat off the flowers. (Plastic screening makes the best strainer because you can squeeze it to remove as much lard as possible.) Repeat the procedure with two more freshly picked batches of flowers before you add alcohol and distill. *Have an adult with you when you do the distillation.* You do not need to remove the last batch of flowers before distillation. If you run into the problem of losing too much fat with each changeover, see how much fragrance you can extract with one or two treatments.

Here are some suggestions for raw materials:

FLOWERS
Roses, carnations, honeysuckle, geranium, gardenias, marigolds

LEAVES
mint, pine needles, bay leaves

FRUITS, NUTS AND BERRIES
ground nutmeg, bayberries, lime peel, ground vanilla bean

BARKS AND ROOTS
ground cinnamon, cedar sawdust

Make sure that any material you select has a strong odor. Faintly smelling flowers do not contain enough essential oils to make extraction worthwhile. You can mix the different extracts to make your own particular perfume. The basic smells of perfumes are: citrus (lemon, lime), florals, mints, spices, woody (cedar, pine needles), fresh green (mowed grass, mashed fresh green peas).

A Study of Perfume

The essential oils that are combined to make perfumes not only smell different from each other, but also evaporate at different rates. This means that once a perfume is exposed to the air, it changes as time passes. You can do a simple experiment to see how a perfume changes over time.

Materials and Equipment
–strips of coffee filter paper ¼ inch wide and about three inches long
–perfume, cologne or after-shave lotion
–clock
–pencil

Procedure
   Dip the end of a strip of filter paper in your perfume sample. Write the time of this activity on the other end of the strip. Set the strip aside.
   After ten minutes, repeat this procedure with a second strip of filter paper. Smell your two strips. Be sure and refresh your nose between sniffs by sniffing your sleeve.
   Repeat your procedure again twenty minutes later. Compare

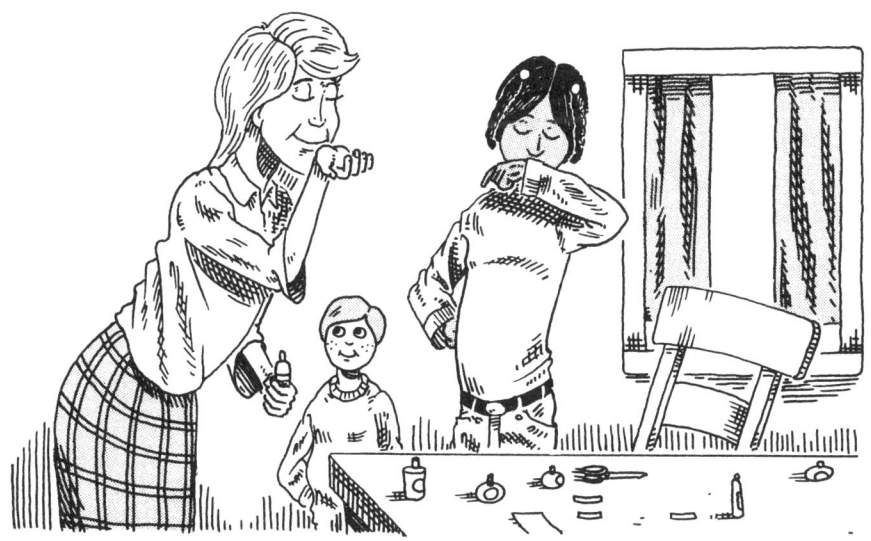

your freshly dipped sample with the one that is now twenty minutes old and one that is thirty minutes old. Make another test one hour after you started, then three hours, or set your own time schedule.

Observations and Suggestions

The aroma you first smell contains the most volatile oils. They are called the "top notes" of a perfume. These oils evaporate first. Just after the top notes have evaporated, the aroma left behind is the "body" of the perfume. The fragrance that remains after several hours is the "dry down." This part of the perfume contains the least volatile oils.

Perfume on your skin behaves differently from perfume on filter paper. Your own skin chemistry mixes with a perfume and alters the smell. Test this idea by sniffing the perfume on the filter paper and perfume on the inside of your wrist.

Perfume on your warm skin also evaporates faster than perfume on filter paper. It evaporates fastest when placed on "pulse points" like the wrist or inside of the elbow, where the blood supply is closest to the surface. Try the time test on your skin. Compare the smells after different time intervals with samples on paper. Compare smells of perfume over a pulse point with perfume placed on the back of your forearm. Experts say that perfume usually lasts about four to six hours on your skin.

One problem is that your nose adjusts to the fine perfume odor as it would to unpleasant odors. After a while you think that the perfume you're wearing has disappeared. It hasn't. You can't smell it any longer, but it's still there.

Perfume Staying Power

Most fine perfumes have ingredients that slow down the rate of evaporation. These are called *fixatives.* A fixative is the least volatile oil and tends to trap the more highly volatile oils. Thus the perfume releases its aroma more slowly.

Years ago one of the fixatives used in fine perfumes was a highly valued substance found floating on the sea called *ambergris.* Ambergris had a slightly sour, salty, seaweedy smell itself and for a while no one knew what it was. Used in very small amounts, it added tremendous warmth to perfumes. It turned out that ambergris was produced by sperm whales. Sperm whales eat squid, a relative of an octopus that has its shell on its inside, like a bone. Since the whale can't digest this shell, its stomach forms a protective coating on it. After it is coated, the whale vomits it up.

Fresh ambergris has a strong, terrible smell. But with aging its smell improves, and it does not interfere with the pleasant smell of a fragrance. Ambergris became so important to the perfume industry that whalers were offered bonuses if they could get it, an added incentive to kill whales. The whaling industry hardly exists anymore, as many whales are now on the endangered species list. Perfume manufacturers can put real ambergris in perfume only if they can prove that it didn't cost the life of a whale. Perfumers now use a synthetic ambergris or other chemicals as fixatives that more than serve this purpose.

Another fixative is musk, a fatty substance from certain male deer. Musk has its own distinctive odor. It is so much less volatile than other fragrances that it doesn't appear to be a very strong odor. Musk perfumes all seem quite weak. They don't have that burst of initial aroma that are the top notes of other perfumes. But they last "forever."

See if you can slow down the rate at which perfume escapes from your skin. Smear some Vaseline over a pulse point on one wrist. Then put perfume over the Vaseline, and put some perfume directly on your skin over the pulse point on your other wrist. Smell them both from time to time. Some of the oils will be held back by the Vaseline, and you should be able to smell this perfume longer than the perfume on your other wrist.

5. Hair

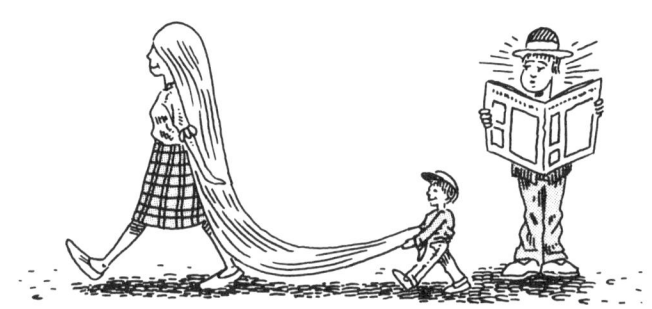

Your skin produces two amazing protective materials, hair and nails, that are both made of exactly the same stuff. At first glance, you might not think this possible, since they appear to be so different. Hair is soft and nails are stiff and tough. Yet, they are both made out of a complicated protein that does not dissolve in water called *hard keratin*. (Soft keratin protects the skin.) The differences between hair and nails are a result of the way hard keratin is structured. Steel wool and a steel plate are both made of the same material, but the structure of the material gives them different qualities.

In certain ways soft hair has its own kind of toughness. Every day it experiences friction as it is brushed and combed. Regular shampooing removes the protective coating of sebum that reduces friction between hairs. Hair can be curled, blown dry, colored, bleached and ironed. And it survives. Most of the hairs on your head are about three years old. The rough treatment has no effect on how long a hair remains attached to your scalp. An average hair lasts two to four years before it falls out to be replaced by a new hair. It is the toughness of hard keratin and the structure of hair that gives hair its remarkable staying power.

Human beings are fairly hairless, compared to other mammals. The hair on fur-covered mammals has the important job of keeping them warm. Each hair has it own tiny muscle that can cause a hair to stand on end. By making hair stand on end, furry animals can trap air, increasing the ability of the fur to maintain body heat. The fine hairs covering our body cannot even begin to do this. Nevertheless, each body hair has its own tiny muscle, a connecting link to our ancestors, who were covered with a coat of hair. When we are cold or frightened, these muscles contract to form "goose bumps," which do very little to keep us warm.

Eyebrow hair protects the eyes by preventing sweat from rolling into them. Eyelashes screen the eyeball from dust in the air. Hair in the nose also traps dust. Hair under the arm reduces friction between the arm and the body. The approximately 100,000 hairs on the head protect the brain from the sun and cushion it against injury. But no matter what its function or its natural length, all hair is produced by hair follicles, and all hair has the same basic structure.

The shaft of a hair is the part that extends above the skin. The root of a hair is the part that lies within the follicle. The bulb of a hair surrounds the papilla. It is made of living cells that have distinct cell boundaries and are filled with liquid. These cells

The hair follicle *is an inward pocket of skin. Each follicle produces one hair, although from two to five hairs may emerge from a single opening on the scalp.*

Papilla—*a conelike growth of the dermis that produces the hair. It is supplied with blood vessels to nourish the growing hair. Baldness and thinning hair are often due to the degeneration of the papillae.*

Sebaceous gland—*manufactures* sebum, *an oily material that lubricates and protects each hair.*

Arrector pili muscle—*a small muscle attached to the wall of a hair follicle and the lower layer of the epidermis. When it contracts, the hair stands on end. It produces "goose bumps." Contraction is triggered by cold or fear.*

Nerve endings—*when a hair is pulled out, these nerves send a message of pain to the brain.*

change as they move up the follicle. By the time they have moved ⅓ of the way, the cell nucleus has died, the cell boundaries have disappeared and chains of hard keratin have linked with each other. The hair now has three separate regions: the *cuticle,* the *cortex* and the *medulla.* Water is now only five percent to ten percent of the weight of a hair. Almost ninety percent of the weight of the cells in the bulb is due to water.

The average person's hair grows at a rate of about ½ inch a month or six to seven inches a year. Most hairs have a maximum length to which they grow. Scalp hair reaches an average length of about two feet, if left uncut. (The world record is six feet one inch.) Some fifty to eighty hairs are shed every day. This means that fifty to eighty new hairs must start growing each day to replace the ones that are shed. Hair follicles don't produce hairs at even rates. Some hairs grow faster than others, so frequent trimming is needed to keep hair length from becoming ragged. The quality of hair is affected by general health and diet. Cutting or shaving has no effect on hair growth.

The chemical properties of hard keratin and the physical properties of hair are constantly being fiddled with in everyone's personal quest for style and good grooming. The experiments in this chapter will introduce you to the properties of hair and nails and the cosmetics we use on them. Since you will be needing samples of hair, I suggest you go to a local hairdresser and ask the staff to save samples of hair for you to experiment with. Ask them to label the samples. Virgin hair has never been treated with chemicals. Hair that has been bleached or permanented is likely to be somewhat damaged.

The Remarkable Hair

Under a microscope, a hair cuticle looks something like fish scales with irregular edges. In healthy, virgin hair, the scales overlap and lie flat against each other. Only the ends of the scales are visible. The cuticle averages between seven and ten scales thick. The ends of the scales point away from the root of the hair. You can feel this. Hold a single hair from your head so that it is taut. Run the thumb and index finger of your other hand back and forth along this hair. Notice that there is no resistance to this motion when moving from the root toward the end. But there is some friction when you move in the opposite direction. That's because your fingers are rubbing against the ends of the cuticle scales. The crinkly sound you hear when you rub hairs together is due to the rough cuticle scales rubbing against each other.

The job of the cuticle is to protect the hair cortex. Its rough surface traps and holds sebum, the oily material produced by the sebaceous glands. Sebum makes hair waterproof and reduces the friction of hairs rubbing against each other. The direction of the scales helps water run off the ends of the hair rather than collect toward the scalp. Tightly layered scales protect the cortex from absorbing too much moisture. Hair that has been treated with strong chemicals often has cuticle scales that are broken and fanned out away from the cortex. Such damaged hair is more *porous;* its surface absorbs water more quickly than healthy, virgin hair. You can see this for yourself. Get two shallow bowls of water. Put a few virgin hairs in one bowl and a few bleached or permanented hairs in the other. The untreated hairs will float. The protective coating on the hair and the tightly packed cuticle scales keep the water from wetting the hair. The hair floats due to surface tension of water in much the same way as a needle can "float" on the surface of water. But the damaged hair will quickly sink, as water is able to wet the hair more quickly.

The cortex makes up from 75 percent to 90 percent of the weight of your hair. It is made of many millions of parallel fibers of hard keratin that are twisted around each other as in a rope. Split ends in damaged hairs are exposed cortex. The cuticle scales at the ends of hairs have broken off. The cortex is responsible for the basic properties of hair. Do the following experiments to explore these properties.

Materials and Equipment
–several hairs about five inches long
–Scotch tape
–keys
–postage balance (optional)
–paper clips
–ruler

Procedure
A healthy, undamaged hair is strong. It should be able to support up to two ounces of weight without breaking. Here's how you can test the strength of a hair. Tape one end of a hair to a towel rack in the bathroom. Stick a paper clip through a key. Pass the free end of the hanging hair through the paper clip to form a loop.

Tape the ends together as shown in the picture. Let the hair hang with the key. Does it break? If it doesn't break, hang a second key on the paper clip. Keep adding keys, one by one, until the hair snaps. Take off the last key you added before the hair snapped. Weigh the keys and paper clip. This weight is slightly less than the weight the hair can support without snapping.

    The length of hair changes when it is wet. Tape a new hair to the towel rack and hang a single key on the end. Measure the exact length of the loop. (Since millimeters are very small units of measurement, you will be most accurate if you measure your hair in millimeters.) Turn on the shower and let the bathroom get all steamed up. Measure the hair again in the steamy bathroom.

Observations and Suggestions

The hairs I tested supported about 1½ ounces before snapping. You can test hairs from different people. Some people will obviously have stronger hair than others. Ask your friends with long hair for samples. Red hair is coarser than black, brown or blond hair. Is it stronger? You'll need to find a friend with long red hair to test this idea. Can you see why human hair has been twisted together into ropes for heavy lifting?

Hair stretches more easily when it is wet. The humidity of the shower should cause the hair to stretch several millimeters. The response of hair to moisture has been used to measure humidity in the air. The instrument that does this is called a "hair hygrometer." Some weather stations use hair hygrometers to measure changes in humidity.

You can use these procedures to compare the differences in hair. How does bleached hair compare to unbleached in strength and elasticity? Curly and straight hair? Blond vs. red vs. brown? Hair from people of different races?

Shampoo, Soap and Conditioners

About 200 years ago, fashionable ladies didn't wash their hair very often. No surprise since they didn't bathe much either. This didn't mean that they didn't build fantastic hairstyles. Eighteenth century France introduced a hairstyle in which long hair was combed straight up from the head over a cushion, where it was fastened with many pins. The back was arranged into hanging curls. Hair was often powdered just before it was arranged, giving it a dull, white look. This kind of elaborate hairstyle was fixed in place for at least three months. Women carried knitting-needlelike instruments to scratch their heads and poke at the insects that lived in their hair. Head lice, insects that can infect the scalp, were common inhabitants of such hairdos.

As people began bathing more often, they started washing their hair also. But not as often as they washed their bodies. Twenty years ago, most well-groomed people washed their hair about once a week. In those days, shampooing hair didn't mean it would instantly look its best. Freshly shampooed hair is slippery and has a lot of "flyaway" or static electricity. Such hair is unmanageable. A typical statement twenty years ago was, "I just washed my hair and I can't do a thing with it." After two days, enough sebum would have been brushed through the hair to make it "behave." After four or five days, the hair started to look greasy from sebum and became stringy as hairs began sticking together. After a week, you couldn't stand it any longer, and a shampoo was in order.

Shampooing removes sweat and dirt from the scalp. It also removes the sebum that protects the hair along with the dirt that sticks to it. Clean hair feels good. Today, people shampoo much more often than they did twenty years ago. Some people wash their hair every day. How do they keep clean hair from being unmanageable? The secret is in hair conditioners.

Do the following experiments to see the effect of soap, shampoo and conditioners on hair.

Materials and Equipment
–cut virgin hair at least three inches long
–small rubber bands
–small dishes
–soap
–knife
–shampoo
–conditioner
–plastic comb with fine teeth

Procedure
Again, the best source of hair for this experiment is your local hairdresser. If you can't get long cut hair for this experiment, you can use the hair on your head. I'll tell you how in a minute.

Make a test tress out of the cut hair. Take a strand of several hundred hairs. Hold them together at one end by twisting a rubber band around them and your finger as in a pony tail. Make the rubber band as tight as possible, then slip your finger from under the rubber band. Make four tresses in all.

Next prepare your test solutions. Use the knife to shave about a teaspoon of soap into one dish. Add enough warm water to make a soapy solution. Put a teaspoon of shampoo into a second dish. Add warm water and stir with your finger. Put one tress into the soap solution and two tresses into the shampoo solution. Stir them with your fingers. Then let them sit for about five minutes. The fourth tress is your control. It should sit in a dish of plain warm water for five minutes.

Rinse each tress well under warm, running water. Be careful to keep track of how each one was treated. Mix about a teaspoon of conditioner in some warm water in a fourth dish. Take one of the tresses that was in shampoo and put it in the conditioner. Stir with your finger, and let it sit there for five minutes. Take it out and rinse it off. Let your tresses dry or blow them dry with a hair dryer.

When your tresses are completely dry, comb them out. Be sure to hold the rubber band end firmly when you comb.

If you want to experiment using the hair on your head, part your hair down the middle from front to back. Pin one side of your hair to hold it out of the way. Alternately, wash one side with soap and the other with shampoo. Rinse well. Divide the side of your hair that was treated with shampoo by parting it from the crown of your head to the back of your ear. Treat the lower portion of hair with conditioner. Rinse. Note: You may have to have a friend help you as it's hard to keep the sections of hair separated.

Observations and Suggestions

Do you see a difference between your hair samples? Although it may be hard to see which shampooed hair is shiniest, it should be obvious that hair washed with soap is the dullest. Soap leaves a film on hair. Shampoo, which contains a detergent, doesn't. An acid rinse is supposed to remove a soap film. Try dipping your soap-treated hair into a dish of lemon juice and water and rinsing again. Does it look shinier when it is dry?

Which tress combs out most easily? If your hair samples are completely dry, and if the day is not hot and humid, you should see "flyaway" as you comb. Which tress exhibits the most flyaway? Which has the least? Comb the tress that has the most flyaway. Bring the comb near the hair but don't let it touch the hair. In which direction does the hair move? Let the hair touch the comb but don't move the comb through the hair. What happens to the flyaway? Stroke the hair with your fingers. What happens to the flyaway?

Here's an explanation of what's happening to your hair. When you comb clean, dry hair, you can make the hairs stand away from each other. This flyaway is an example of a material that has become *charged* due to static electricity. Static electricity acts like a magnet. It can attract or repel other charged objects. You've seen it attract objects when you remove clothes from the dryer that are sticking to each other. Both the hair and the comb are charged with static electricity. Hairs move away from each other and toward the comb. This demonstrates two very important aspects of static electricity:

1. There are two kinds of static electrical charges. One is called *negative* and the other is called *positive*.

2. Opposite charges attract each other. The comb and hair have opposite charges. Similar charges repel each other. Flyaway is caused by all the hairs having a similar charge. Thus they fly away from each other. Combs made of different materials can cause the hairs to become either positive or negative. But in each case the hairs will repel each other.

Static electricity is caused by a change in the distribution of negatively charged particles, called *electrons,* that exist in the atoms of all matter. Matter also contains positively charged particles. Normally, the number of positive and negative charges in a material is the same. When the charges in a material are balanced, it has no overall charge and is electrically neutral. When a hair becomes electrically charged by combing, you are rubbing electrons from the hair onto the comb, or adding electrons to the hair from the comb. In both cases, you are changing the balance of electrons, and both hair and comb become charged. When you touch the comb to the hair or run your fingers over the hair, the electron balance is restored, and you have "discharged" the static electricity.

Hair conditioners may contain lanolin, fat from sheep that is similar to sebum. This restores some of the protection against dryness that is lost by frequent shampooing. It contains substances that also make hair easier to comb and reduce the damage caused by combing out tangles. Hair conditioners also contain chemicals that are like fabric softeners and reduce the static electricity of flyaway. Do your observations confirm these facts?

Curl

Some people have naturally curly hair and some people have straight hair. The experts aren't sure what causes hair to be naturally curly. Some say that curly hair is caused by the shape of the hair shaft. A round cross section is straight hair, an oval cross section is curly and a flattened cross section is very curly. Another idea is that the shape of the follicle determines the shape of the

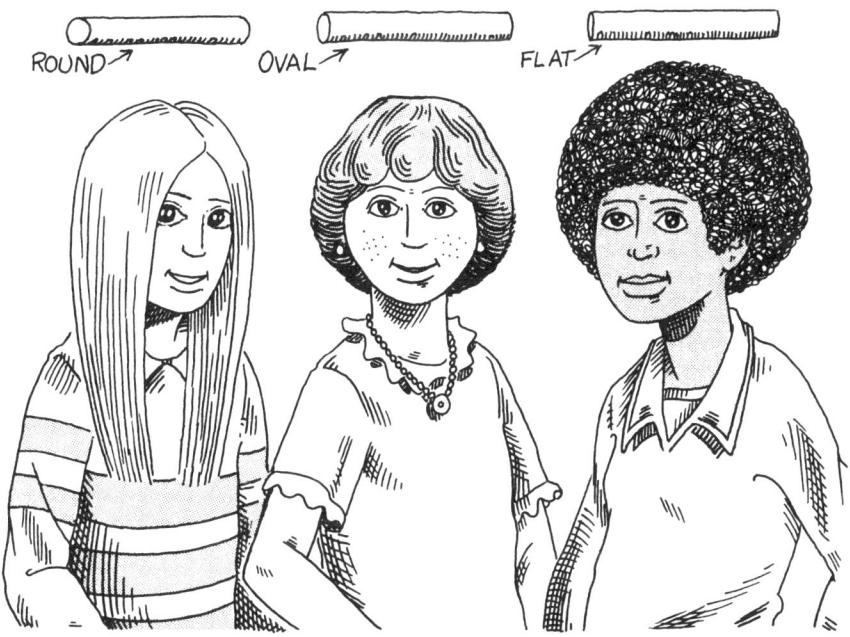

hair. The hair cells are soft when they first form. They could harden to take the shape of the follicle as they grow out. Still another theory is that the papilla decides curl. If hair cells are produced evenly, hair should be straight. If one side of the papilla produces hair cells faster than the other, hair will grow in curves. No one is quite sure yet what causes naturally curly hair. But there's no problem making a curl artificially.

The hard keratin chains in the cortex are held in place by a weak attraction between hydrogen atoms that stick out from the surface of the hard keratin molecules. These *hydrogen bonds* also hold the hair in its natural form, straight or curly. Since the hydrogen bonds are weak, they are easily broken by softening the hair with water or setting lotion. After softening, if the hair is wound in a pin curl or around a roller and allowed to dry, new hydrogen bonds form holding the hair in the new position. That's what setting hair is all about. As set hair absorbs moisture from the air, these new hydrogen bonds are quickly broken, and the hair returns to its natural state. Straight, again. There is no damage to hair that is curled by changing only the hydrogen bonds.

The ability to form hydrogen bonds is temporarily affected by treatment of hair with water, shampoos, soaps and hair conditioners. You can design experiments to see what kind of curl you get in hair samples that have had different treatment. Simply make pincurls the same size in your hair sample tresses, let them dry and comb them out. Does clean hair make a better curl than unclean? Does a waving solution make a difference? Can you curl dry hair? Experiment and find out.

Permanent Waves

Like all proteins, hard keratin is made up of chains of smaller molecules called *amino acids*. All amino acids contain the elements carbon, hydrogen, oxygen and nitrogen. A few kinds of amino acids also contain atoms of sulfur, and these sulfur-containing amino acids are responsible for the shape of a hair. Two sulfur atoms on neighboring amino acids form a strong chemical bond that can be broken only with a chemical reaction. These sulfur bonds maintain the shape of a hair. A chemical reaction with these bonds is the basis for a permanent wave.

When someone gets a permanent wave, the hair is first shampooed, assuring that the hair is thoroughly wet and that the hydrogen bonds are broken. Second, the hair is wound on curlers called "rods" and treated with a chemical that breaks down the sulfur bonds. This makes the hair very soft. Third, the hair is rinsed while it is still on the rods. Fourth, it is treated with a second chemical that "neutralizes" the waving lotion by causing new sulfur bonds to form. These new bonds permanently hold the hair in its curly shape.

The curl produced by a permanent reconnects only about half of the sulfur bonds broken by the waving solution. Treated hair is never as strong as it was originally, and in time the hair relaxes toward its natural shape. Since a permanent wave doesn't affect newly grown hair, it has to be repeated to keep the curly look. Too much permanent waving can severely damage hair.

The chemicals in home permanent wave kits can be purchased in any pharmacy. If you wish to experiment as a scientist with home permanents on *cut* hair tresses, the purchase of a kit is worth the investment. You can try the waving solution for different periods of time. You can try the waving solution on different kinds of hair. *Note: the chemicals in permanent wave kits are strong and poisonous. Don't experiment with them without having an adult present. Do not use on your own hair. Read and follow package directions carefully.*

Bleaching Hair

Hair color is caused by a pigment called *melanin*. Melanin is found in tiny round bodies or *granules* inside the hair cortex. The melanin granules can be tightly packed or grouped in clusters.

They can contain different amounts of pigment. Melanin comes in four colors: black, brown, yellow and red. Most people have a mixture of two or more different pigments in their hair. Air spaces in the cortex also change the overall look of hair color. Gray hair is caused by a loss of pigment. There is no color in the hair cuticle.

A popular way of changing natural hair color is to make it lighter. Hair can be bleached by the sun. This effect is interesting because the sun's rays have the opposite effect on the melanin in the skin. The sun's rays cause an increase in production of melanin in the skin, so the skin gets darker (you get a tan), while melanin in hair is destroyed, so hair gets lighter.

Do the next experiment to see how chemicals can dissolve melanin to produce lighter hair. Will laundry bleach lighten hair? Experiment and be surprised. *Note: The chemicals used to bleach the sample tresses of hair are poisonous. Have an adult with you when doing this experiment.*

Materials and Equipment
–3 sample tresses of brown or black virgin hair
–3 dishes
–measuring spoons
–liquid chlorine bleach (poison)
–hydrogen peroxide (3% solution from a pharmacy)
–ammonia (poison)

Procedure
Do not do any of this procedure to the hair on your head, as

it can cause permanent damage. Use only sample tresses of hair.

Put three tablespoons of liquid bleach in one dish, three tablespoons of hydrogen peroxide in each of the two other dishes. Put ½ teaspoon ammonia in one dish of hydrogen peroxide. Put a tress of hair in each dish and make sure that they become thoroughly wet with the solution. Let them sit for several hours in a well-ventilated area.

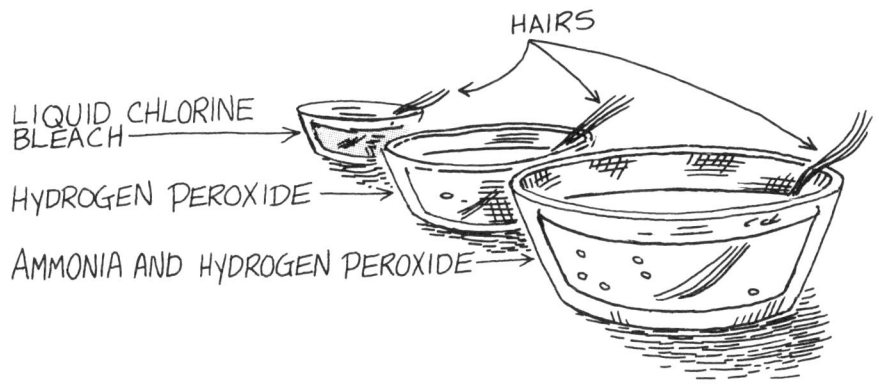

Observations and Suggestions

Hydrogen peroxide is an unstable compound that breaks down into oxygen and water. If you hold a sample of hydrogen peroxide in a glass up to the light, you can see tiny bubbles of oxygen gas rising to the surface. When the oxygen in hydrogen peroxide reaches the melanin granules, it reacts with or *oxidizes* the melanin. The newly produced *oxymelanin* has a red or yellow color and the hair is lighter. As your experiment shows, hydrogen peroxide alone will not do the job. Hydrogen peroxide must be in the presence of a strong base, like ammonia, in order to work. The ammonia swells the cuticle and the hair so that the hydrogen peroxide can enter and react with the melanin.

To stop the bleaching process, it is not enough just to rinse all the ammonia and hydrogen peroxide off the hair. Hair should also be given an acid rinse to neutralize the ammonia and allow the cuticle to shrink back to its normal size. You can see this in another experiment. Bleach two samples of hair. Rinse one sample under water and allow it to dry. Rinse the other sample under water, then dip it in some white vinegar (acid). Rinse off the vinegar and allow it to dry. Do the two bleached samples have different textures? The hair that was not treated with acid should feel coarser and drier.

Did the chlorine bleach lighten the hair? Surprise! The chlorine bleach completely dissolved the hair. Like hydrogen peroxide, chlorine bleach is also an "oxidizer," but it is much stronger than the peroxide. Oxidizers will react first with melanin, but they will also react with the sulfur bonds in the hard keratin, breaking them down. When bleaching is controlled, it is stopped after it has oxidized the melanin but before it can damage the hard keratin. In the experiment the fibers are completely destroyed and the hair dissolves. Chlorine in swimming pools is much more diluted, but it can lighten and dry out hair if the hair is exposed to it often enough.

A warning on the chlorine bleach bottle says that it should not be used on wool or silk. Wool and silk are both fibers made by animals. They are similar to hair. What do you suppose this bleach would do to these fabrics?

6. Makeup

Who doesn't want to be good-looking? No one, that's for sure. And if the shape of your face or nose or mouth doesn't make you a beauty, you still can have striking eyes with thick lashes, rosy cheeks, red lips and teeth as white as possible. Cosmetics can help by adding color, hiding blemishes and accenting the positive.

Makeup is definitely a fashion that changes with the times. People all over the world, from ancient times to the present, have decorated their faces and bodies with paint. The first face and body painters were not so much interested in being beautiful as in pleasing the gods. But Cleopatra, the beautiful queen of Ancient Egypt who lived about 2,000 years ago, may have been the first to set a trend in the use of eye makeup. Cleopatra painted her eyes with *kohl,* a black, green or blue powder containing the element *antimony.* Antimony compounds may be colored and are used as pigments. Cleopatra put black kohl on her upper eyelids and more kohl on her eyelashes. She painted the areas just under her eyes green or blue. Poppaea, the beautiful wife of Nero, the cruel Roman emperor who ruled almost 2,000 years ago, painted her face white with a mixture of white lead and grease. Cleopatra and Poppaea were among the first of a long line of royal women who set the standards for beauty and fashion of their day.

If you go to museums and look at pictures of women through the ages, you can get a sense of the many different kinds of "looks" people have found beautiful. Sometimes a pale look was in, other times rosy cheeks and lips were preferred. In the Middle Ages, women plucked out their eyebrows and eyelashes and shaved their hairlines, giving their faces a bald and uninteresting appearance by today's standards. Queen Elizabeth I, who lived in the sixteenth century, dyed her hair red, or wore red wigs, and powdered her face white. Elizabethan women covered skin blemishes with patches cut from black satin in many different shapes. The favorites were stars, crescents and diamonds. At one time, a silhouette of a coach and horses was a popular patch for the forehead. Makeup became so extreme that by the eighteenth century, the British Parliament passed a law saying that if a woman used "perfume, paints, artificial teeth, wigs . . ." to get a husband, the marriage could be annulled, and she could be convicted of witchcraft.

America, in the eighteenth century, was influenced by the Puritans, who believed the use of makeup was sinful. Actresses in the eighteenth and nineteenth centuries wore makeup to make their features easier to see and more expressive when they were viewed from a distance. In fact, the word "makeup" came from the theater, where actors and actresses "made up" their faces before a performance. Actresses' use of makeup often added to the general opinion that they must, therefore, be women of low moral standards. Nice girls might pinch their cheeks and bite their lips but they never (horrors!), but never, painted their faces.

The American attitude toward makeup began changing at the beginning of the twentieth century. By 1920, lipstick and rouge were acceptable as long as their use wasn't obvious. Slowly, more daring women started using eye makeup and nail polish. But

World War II was the clincher. It was a grim time, and makeup was an inexpensive way for women to give themselves a small treat. Although there were many shortages during the war, it was unthinkable to stop manufacturing lipstick. At the end of the war, the cosmetics industry exploded. Inexpensive and safe makeup was widely available.

In this chapter, you'll explore the properties of the most common types of makeup. *One word of warning. Some people have allergic reactions to substances they put on their skin. Some of the cosmetics you'll be creating are made of materials not intended to be used as makeup. They are not dangerous, but you may have an allergic reaction to them. I've included these recipes because they are fun to make and try. But they are not intended for prolonged use or replacement of commercially available cosmetics that have been backed by extensive laboratory testing. To be extra careful, test your makeup on the backs of your hands, not on your face.*

Powder

One way of covering the skin is to coat it with powder, a soft, finely divided material. At one time or another, most white powders, including flour and cornstarch, have been used as cosmetics. Neither flour nor cornstarch is particularly satisfactory. Flour absorbs moisture and cakes up. Prolonged use of cornstarch can clog pores and cause pimples.

One of the most widely used powders back in Elizabethan days was *ceruse*, a white compound of lead, carbon and oxygen. It was used in abundance to powder the faces of women and the hair of both men and women. Some people had "powder rooms" in their homes, where they could dust themselves freely without worrying that the powder would fly all over everything. Much of the ceruse used in England was imported from Holland. The Dutch were masters of manufacturing fine pigments, and the best ceruse was made there. (Dutch pigments were also used in oil paint. So it's no surprise that the some of the world's finest painters also came from Holland.) In those days there was no agency like the FDA or OSHA to protect consumers and workers against the harmful effects of a cosmetic. The workmen who made ceruse suffered stomach cramps, constipation, shortness of breath, dizziness, severe headaches and even blindness, all symptoms of lead poisoning. No doubt some of its users also were affected. But vanity won out over health until a better powder was made available—a mineral called *talc.*

Talc is a compound of magnesium, silicon, and oxygen. It is an extremely stable substance and will not interact chemically with your skin. But its main advantage as a skin powder is that it is very soft and somewhat slippery. Thus powder made from talc has a silky feel, and powder grains cling to each other and to your skin, making a smooth coating. In nature, talc may be white, gray or green. For the purposes of cosmetics, only the white mineral is used. As a cosmetic, it is known as talcum powder.

Baby powder is often a pure talcum powder product. It may contain only talc and some perfume. Other talcum powders may contain zinc stearate, which acts to make the particles of powder cling even more closely to each other and to spread more easily on the skin, and other additives. Talcum powders for the body are usually white. But face powders must be tinted if they are going to give the face a smooth, even skin tone.

Do the following experiment to make different kinds of face powders.

Materials and Equipment
–cornstarch
–baby talcum powder
–colored, nontoxic chalk (red or pink)
–plastic bags
–hammer or rolling pin
–two nesting steel mixing bowls or a metal bowl and a large tablespoon
–yellow and red food coloring
–custard cup
–spoon
–cotton balls

Procedure
There are two basic parts to your face powders, the powder base and the pigment or coloring material. There are no hard and fast rules here for making your face powder. I'll give you proportions I used in my kitchen, but you can mix your own shades. There are two things to keep in mind. First, your pigment must be ground as fine as possible and be as even in texture as you can make it. Second, the powder base and the pigment must be thoroughly mixed, so that the face powder is not streaky.

Make a powder of cornstarch and chalk. Wrap a piece of colored chalk in a plastic bag. Smash it with the side of your hammer or pound it with a rolling pin. Be careful not to break the bag, or you will lose some of your pigment. Put the smashed chalk into a metal bowl. You are now going to grind it as fine as possible. The usual equipment for hand grinding is a *mortar* and *pestle*.

Normally, this is a stone or wooden bowl (the mortar) and a blunt, rounded tool (the pestle) that you lean on and rotate against the material in the mortar. In the old days, every kitchen had a mortar and pestle for grinding spices and herbs. But today, we often buy our spices already ground, and not every kitchen has a mortar and pestle. So you have to improvise. Since you will be putting pressure on your "pestle," you should not try to grind your pigment in a glass or china bowl that can break, or in a plastic bowl that is soft and will become pitted and scarred by your grinding operation. I found that two nesting steel mixing bowls are ideal. You put the smashed chalk in the larger bowl. Then you crush it with the bottom of the smaller bowl, leaning on your hand and turning the smaller bowl against the chalk. Every once in a while, lift up the smaller bowl and scrape off anything that clings to it, and stir up your pigment. Then go back to your crushing motion. If you don't have two bowls, you can grind pigment by pressing and rubbing the pigment against the side of a metal bowl with the back of a spoon.

When the chalk is powdered and even, mix it with cornstarch. You can mix it with a spoon in a dish, or you can put it in a plastic bag and shake it until the pigment is evenly spread throughout the white powder.

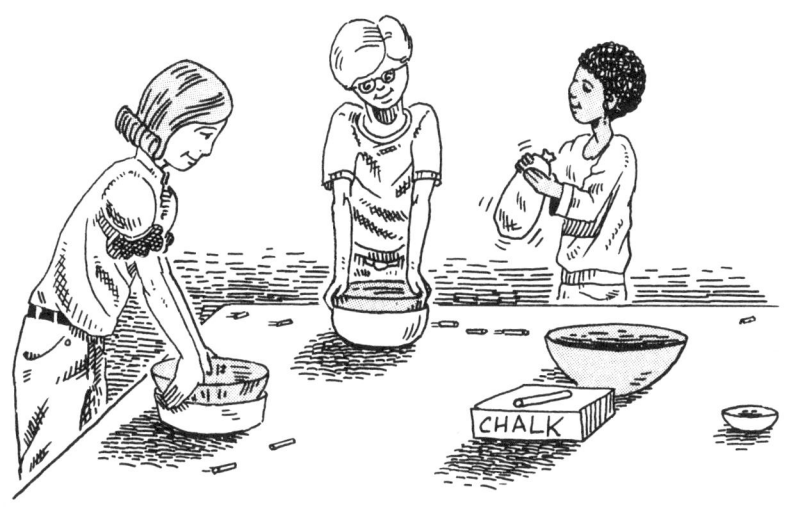

    To make a talc-based face powder, put about a tablespoon of baby talcum powder in a custard cup. Add four drops of red food coloring and three drops of yellow. Notice that the drops remain intact, they don't wet the talcum powder. Mix the food coloring and talcum powder together. At first, the drops will stick in one place, but if you press the powder against the side of the cup with a spoon, as if you were grinding the powder, the food coloring will eventually spread throughout the powder, making quite a nice face powder. Make sure that you mix the food coloring well, or your powder will put red and yellow streaks on your skin. If the powder coloring is too strong, add more talcum.

    Try your face powder on the back of your hand. Apply by dipping a cotton ball in the powder and patting the ball on your hand. To compare the two powders, put some on one hand and some on the other.

Observations and Suggestions

Which powder feels smoother? Which feels drier? Which is the better coverup? How do your homemade powders compare to commercial face powder? What happens if you color cornstarch with food coloring? Color talcum with chalk? Add a few drops of mineral oil to your powder and work it in with a spoon. What happens to the texture?

Suppose you make your talcum powder a bright red. Could you use it as rouge? Experiment and find out. A word of warning. The water in food coloring, which you mixed with talc, can attract certain bacteria, so this powder can eventually spoil and perhaps cause problems on your skin. *The powders in this experiment are not meant for use over a long period of time.*

Powder "Wetting" Test

Different powders have different abilities to absorb oil. This factor is important to cosmetic manufacturers because oily skin can cause a powder to cake up. The next experiment shows you how to test a powder for its "wetting" ability, the amount of oil it can absorb before becoming a paste.

Materials and Equipment
–cornstarch
–talcum powder
–mineral oil
–measuring spoons
–2 custard cups

–2 butter knives
–straw or eye dropper
–2 teaspoons

Procedure

Put ½ level teaspoon of cornstarch in one custard cup. To make a level teaspoon, run the back of a knife over the ½ teaspoon that is overfilled with powder. Put ½ level teaspoon of talcum in the other cup. Wash and dry the measuring spoon before measuring out the talcum and use a different knife to make it level.

Add a drop of oil to each powder. If you have an eye dropper, it is easy to measure drops. If not, a straw works quite well. Use the straw as a chemist uses an instrument called a *pipette.* Dip the straw in the oil. Put your index finger over the top of the straw as you remove the straw from the oil. The oil will remain in the straw. If you carefully bend the first knuckle of your index finger backwards by pressing down on it, you can let in a tiny amount of air. In this way, you can release one drop of oil at a time. It takes a little practice to get control, but this is a skill that most chemists develop.

Work the drop of oil into each sample by rubbing it with the back of the spoon. Keep working drops of oil into each powder, a drop at a time, making sure that you keep an accurate count. The number of drops needed to turn the oil into a paste is a measure of the tendency of a powder to absorb oil.

Observations and Suggestions

A paste forms from a powder when the powder grains are

coated with oil and can stick together. I found that the cornstarch formed a paste after eight drops and the talcum formed a paste with ten drops.

Repeat the experiment with water instead of oil. Which kind of powder should remain longer on the skin without caking up due to the absorption of either water or oil from the skin?

Lipstick

Lipstick, as we know it today, came into use just before World War I. All lipsticks, from then to the present, contain an oil-wax base and two kinds of coloring agents, *dyes* and *pigments.* A dye dissolves in the base and will stain the lips. Dyes are the basis for long-lasting lipsticks, which were popular in the 1950s and are currently coming back in style. Pigments do not dissolve but are suspended in a base. Pigments are not absorbed by the skin but stick to its surface. A pigment's ability to color something depends on how densely and evenly it is distributed in the base, and this depends on how finely it is ground. Pigments that are used in cosmetics and paints are ground in mills. For this reason, they are called *milled pigments.*

Milled pigments that are already suspended in a wax base are found in crayons. You can make your own lip gloss out of a crayon.

Materials and Equipment
–beeswax (a beeswax candle is the source that's easiest to find)
–mineral oil
–$3\tfrac{5}{8}$ inch $\times$ $\tfrac{5}{16}$ inch nontoxic crayon

–measuring spoons
–heat resistant custard cup
–plastic bag
–hammer
–paper toweling
–small saucepan
–knife
–spoon for stirring

Procedure

Put about one teaspoon beeswax in the custard cup. This is a ½ inch slice of a beeswax candle one inch in diameter. Add three tablespoons mineral oil to the cup. Put the crayon in a plastic bag, and smash it with a hammer. This makes it easy to remove the paper wrapper. Put the smashed crayon in the cup.

Set the custard cup in the small saucepan that contains enough water to reach a level of about 1½ inches up the side of the custard cup. *Check with an adult before you use the stove.* Put the setup over a medium heat. Heat, stirring occasionally, until the waxes are melted and the color is evenly spread throughout the liquid. Turn off the heat and allow your lip gloss to cool for five to ten minutes.

Observations and Suggestions

When you apply your lip gloss to the back of your hand, it will look quite shiny. This is due to the oil in the base. The beeswax stiffens the mixture and holds the pigment. The combination of wax and oil, which mix evenly with each other when hot, produces a base that is still soft enough to spread easily. The milled pigments are carried along by the base.

You can use the custard cup in a water bath to make recycled lipsticks out of old lipsticks your mother may have around the house. As always, check with an adult before using the stove. Put the old lipsticks in the cup, melt them in the water bath, mix thoroughly and create new shades.

When you test your creations, try them out on the back of your hand. If you can see through them, they are *translucent* or *transparent.* If they make a strong color that you can't see through, they are *opaque.* If they have a "frosted" look they probably contain ground fish scales or ground synthetic pearls.

About Nails

In the past, the length of one's fingernails was an indication of social class. People who work with their hands cannot have long, well-shaped fingernails. They would get in the way. So long nails sent a message that the wearer was a person of leisure, someone who could afford not to work with his or her hands. (Of course, many women do manage to have long fingernails in spite of the fact that they use their hands for activities that are hard on nails.) Historically, women have not been the only ones to grow their nails. Certain ancient Chinese noblemen grew such long fingernails that they literally could do nothing for themselves. Servants had to dress them, feed them and bathe them.

According to the *Guinness Book of World Records,* the longest fingernail ever grown was 25½ inches long, grown over a period of thirteen years by Romesh Sharma of Delhi, India. It was measured in 1979. The longest set of nails belonged to the left hand of Shridhar Chillal, also of India. The five nails were measured in 1984 and had been growing uncut since 1952. The total length was 135 inches (the thumbnail was thirty-two inches). Naturally his nails had not been manicured and they curled as they grew. I have no idea if he treated them to prevent them from breaking.

 Fingernails and toenails are produced by cells at the base of the nail called the *nail matrix*. The actual nail is called the *nail plate*. The cells that form in the matrix are pushed forward to form the nail plate. As they grow, they die and lose the boundaries between them, forming many layers of hard keratin. It takes between 117 and 138 days for a cell to move from the matrix to the fingertip. The *nail bed* lies under the nail plate and attaches the nail plate to the finger. It is made up of living cells that move forward with the nail plate. If the nail bed is injured, it may separate from the nail plate, and eventually the nail plate will be lost as a new nail forms beneath it. The half-moon, or *lunula,* at the base of the nail is the visible part of the matrix which extends beneath the skin of the finger. The nail *cuticle* is the frame of mostly dead skin surrounding the nail plate. If left uncut or pushed back, it will grow over part of the nail forming a tight covering that can split, causing "hangnails." Since hangnails can become infected, it's a good idea to keep cuticles softened with creams and pushed back against the skin.

A manicure keeps the cuticles trimmed and gives the ends of the nails an even edge that is free of splits and cracks. Whether you have long or short nails, it's a good idea to make sure that you have no rough edges, which can be extremely annoying when they catch on things.

Nail Polish

A manicure typically involves painting the nails with nail polish. The ancient Egyptians colored nails with dyes, but nail enamel, as we know it, has only been around since the early 1920s. Nail enamel is made up of the following ingredients:

Milled pigments—finely ground, insoluble material that is suspended in the base.

Nitrocellulose—this is a plastic film-forming material that is made by boiling wood pulp in sulfuric and nitric acid. Wood pulp contains fibers of *cellulose.* The manufacturing process adds nitrates to the cellulose chains. The addition of nitrates now allows the cellulose chains to interlock and form a film, the basis for the enamel coating. Nitrocellulose is used for nail enamel because it wears well, it bonds fairly well to the nail, it is somewhat glossy, and most importantly, it allows the nail to "breathe." No matter how many coats you put on your fingernails, moisture and gases can pass through the film. If this didn't happen, skin fungus could grow under the film, causing all kinds of problems.

Solvent—this is a liquid that dissolves the nitrocellulose, and when it evaporates, the film forms. Without a solvent, you could not spread the nail enamel on your nails.

Plasticizer—nitrocellulose makes a fairly brittle film. A plasticizer is an additive that keeps the film flexible. However, in time, the plasticizer ages and eventually nail polish will chip.

Suspending agent—this is an ingredient that keeps the pigment evenly spread throughout the liquid. Most nail polish needs to be shaken before use because some of the heavier pigment particles tend to settle. But without a suspending agent, all the pigment would settle within twenty-four hours, and you would have clear liquid on top.

Do the following experiment to investigate nail polish.

Materials and Equipment
- nail polishes of different brands (whatever you have around your house)
- Saran Wrap
- aluminum foil
- waxed paper
- 3 rubber bands
- 3 jars or cups
- scissors

Procedure

Stretch the Saran Wrap over the mouth of a jar or cup and hold it in place with the rubber band. It should have a smooth, taut surface. Do the same thing with the waxed paper and the aluminum foil.

Paint a spot of each nail polish sample on each surface. Let them dry.

Observations and Suggestions

The nail polish you put on Saran Wrap seems to sink into it. This indicates that the polish is a plastic that dissolves into Saran Wrap, a similar plastic film.

The nail polish on the foil forms a film. If you make several applications to form a thick film, you may be able to peel the dried film from the foil.

The polish on the waxed paper doesn't seem to dry. Nail polish has a "drying time," usually less than an hour, and a "setting time," a slow hardening of the polish. This takes about twelve hours. The reason the polish doesn't dry on the waxed paper is that the solvent in the polish dissolves some of the wax. Wax acts as a plasticizer, combining with the solvent and preventing it from evaporating.

The Proof of the Pudding...

No matter how much a scientist in the cosmetics industry may test products for safety and quality in the laboratory, there comes a time when a product must be tested by potential users. Nail polish is not intended for coating household wraps. It's supposed to put gloss and color on your fingernails. Here's how nail polish manufacturers test their products against their competition.

Since you use different fingers different amounts and one hand more than the other, paint every other finger of both hands with one brand of nail polish. Then paint the unpainted fingernails with a second brand of polish. If you don't want to look strange, try to match the colors. But if you don't care, use different colors so you keep track of which brand is which. Put on at least two coats. As you wear the polish, watch for peeling (caused by moisture collecting under the polish) and chipping, caused by too little plasticizer.

One final word . . . Although you have been investigating cosmetics scientifically in this book, science is only a part of the secret life of cosmetics. Some are designed to keep you clean and healthy. Others are products that are meant to be enjoyed. The personal use of cosmetics is not a science but an art . . . one that you may have the great pleasure of discovering for yourself.

Appendix

The essential oils listed below can be found at specialty shops for extracts and flavorings.

Recipe for "Pure Joy"

Heliotropin	30 drops
Oil of rose	1⅞ tsp
Synthetic bergamot oil	60 drops
Musk	4 drops
Ambergris	12 drops
Artificial jasmine	12 drops
Neroli oil	4 drops
Angelica	8 drops
Vetivert	8 drops
Medium perfume oil base	3 fluid ounces

Blend all the ingredients. Yield: approximately 3½ ounces.

Index

Page numbers in *italic* refer to illustrations.

acids, 18–21
advertising, 3
alkali, 18–21
ambergris, 64–65
amino acids, 80
ammonia, 83, *83*, 84
antimony, 86
arrector pili muscle, 68, *68*
atoms, 16
attar, 56

baby powder, 90
bacteria, 21–24
bases, 18–21
bathing, history of, 7–10
beauty secrets, 3–6
bed, nail, 99
beeswax, 40, 41, 96, 97

bleach, liquid chlorine, 83, *83*, 84–85
bleaching, hair, 81–85, *83*
body of perfume, 63
borax, 40, 41, *42*

calluses, 31, 32
Castile soap, 12
cellulose, 100
ceruse, 89–90
chlorine bleach, liquid, 83, *83*, 84–85
Cleopatra and makeup, 86–87
cold cream, 40–44, *42*
collagen, 33
condenser, 58, *58*, 60
conditioners, hair, 74–78
connective tissue, 33

controls in experiments, 16
cornstarch, 4, 89, 92, 94–96
cortex, hair, 69
cosmetic cream, 36–40
  experiments with, 37–40, *38*
cosmetics
  definition of, 4
  history of, 4–5
  See also makeup.
curl, 78–80, *79*
cuticles,
  hair, 69
  nails, 100

dentifrices, 25–27
deodorant soaps, 21–24
dermis, 31
detergent, 14–15, 17, 19
distillation of essential oils, 56–60, *58*
dry down of perfume, 63
dyes in lipstick, 96

Edelweiss perfume, 54–55
electrons, 78
element, 16
emollient, 44
emulsifiers, 36
emulsion stability test, 44–45
emulsions, 36
enfleurage, 56
epidermis, 31

epsom salt, 13
essential oils
  extraction of, 55–62, *58*
  Pure Joy recipe, 105
eyebrow hair, 67
eyelashes, 67

fatty acid chain, 17
fingernails, 98–100
fixatives, perfume, 64–65
flour, 89
fluoride, 26–27
follicles, hair, 67, 68–69, *68*
Food and Drug Administration (FDA), 32, 90
fragrances, 46–65
  and sense of smell, 46–52, *51*
  and the triangle test, 49–52, *51*

gels, 33
gelatin, 33
  test, 33–36, *35*
goose bumps, 31, 67, 68

hair, 66–85
  bleaching of, 81–85, *83*
  conditioners for, 74–78
  cortex of, 70, 71
  curl of, 78–80, *79*
  cuticle of, 70
  length of, 72–73
  permanent waves in, 80–81

rate of growth of, 69
regions of, 69
structure of, 67–69, *68*
test for strength of, 71–73, *72*
washing of, 73–74
hair hygrometers, 73
half-moons, 100
hangnails, 100
hydrogen bonds, 79–80, 81
hydrogen peroxide, 83–84, *83*

indicator dyes, 18

keratin, hard, 66, 69, 71
  chains, 79
kohl, 86–87
kosmetikos, 3
kosmos, 3

lanolin, 78
lead poisoning, 90
lipstick, 96–98
litmus tests, 18
lotions, 36–40
lunulas, 100
lye, 12, 18

makeup, 86–103
  history of, 86–89
  lipstick, 96–98
  nails, 98–100
  powder, 89–96

manicures, 100
matrix, nail, 99
market testing, 39–40
medulla, hair, 69
melanin, 81–82
  granules, 81–82
milled pigments, 96–98, 100
molds, 23
molecules, 16–17
mortar and pestle, 92
musk, 65

nails, 98–100
  structure of, 99
nail polish, 100–102
nerve endings, 68, *68*
nitrocellulose, 100–101

oil, skin, 94–96
oil-in-water (O/W) emulsions, 36–37
olfactory nerve, 47
oxidizers, 83–84
oxymelanin, 83

papilla, 67, 68, *68*
perfume, 52–66
  basic smells of, 62
  definition of, 52
  dry down of, 63
  history of, 52–53
  staying power of, 64–65

perfume (cont.)
   study of, 62–64, *63*
   top notes of, 63
permanent waves, 80–81
pH, 20–21
phenolphthalein, 18
pigments, milled, 96–98, 100
pipette, 95
plasticizer, 101
plate, nail, 99
Poppaea, 87
pores, 31
powder, 89–96
   "wetting" test, 94–96
powder rooms, 90
public baths, 8–9
pulse points, 64
Pure Joy perfume, 54–55, 105

Roman baths, 8–9

salt, 18–19
sample, 39–40
sebaceous glands, 31, 68, *68*
sebum, 16, 31, 68, 70, 74
shampoo, 73–78
skin, 30–32
   cells of, 31
   function of, 30–32
smell, 46–49
   definition of, 46
   triangle test, 49–52, *51*

soap, 10–24
   Castile, 12
   chemistry of, 11–12
   history of, 10–12
soapmaking in Colonial America, 12
soap molecules, 16–17, *17*
solvents, 101
sperm whales, 64–65
static electricity, 77–78
   charges, 77–78
statistics, 39–40
stratum corneum, 31, 32–33
sulfur bonds, 80–81
suspending agent, 101
sweat glands, 31

talc, 90
talcum powder, 90–91, 94–96
teeth, 24–29
   and appearance, 24
toothcare, 24–27
tooth decay, 27
toothpaste, 26
   test, 27–29
toothpicks, 26
top notes of perfume, 63
triangle test, 49–52

Vaseline, 34, 35
Vaughan's Water, 25–26
virgin hair, 69, 70

water, hard, 12
water-in-oil (W/O) emulsions, 36–37
waves, permanent, 80–81

William Colgate & Company, 26

zinc stearate, 90

About the Author

Vicki Cobb earned her bachelor's degree from Barnard College and received a master's degree from Columbia University's Teachers College.

After an early career as a science teacher, Ms. Cobb turned to writing. In addition to many award-winning books for young people, she has written scripts for network television and was the creator and host of *The Science Game,* an educational TV series. She now divides her time between writing and speaking to children, teachers, and librarians all over the country.

About the Illustrator

Theo Cobb has been drawing since he was two years old, and won a New York City art contest when he was five. He attends the School of Visual Arts in New York City. The first book he illustrated was CHEMICALLY ACTIVE, also by his mother, Vicki Cobb.